Molecular Biology
Biochemistry and Biophysics
15

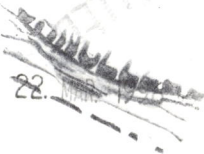

Mitchel Weissbluth

Hemoglobin

Cooperativity and Electronic Properties

With 50 Figures

Chapman & Hall Limited · London

Springer-Verlag Berlin · Heidelberg · New York 1974

Professor Dr. M. WEISSBLUTH

Department of Applied Physics
and
W. W. Hansen Laboratories of Physics
Standford University
Stanford, CA 94305/USA

ISBN 0-412-12840-3 Chapman & Hall Ltd. London

ISBN 3-540-06582-2 Springer-Verlag Berlin Heidelberg New York
ISBN 0-387-06582-2 Springer-Verlag New York Heidelberg Berlin

Preface

Approximately one third of the mass of a mammalian red blood cell is hemoglobin. Its major function is to bind oxygen at the partial pressure prevailing in the lungs and to release it to the tissues where the partial pressure is lower. The process whereby hemoglobin performs this essential physiological role is characterized by a cooperative interaction among its constituent subunits. A great deal of research effort has been devoted to this interaction, going back at least as far as the first decade of this century. Moreover, cooperativity in hemoglobin is probably not unique; it may well be one instance of a general class of interactions that occur in biological molecules. Certain enzymes with a variety of regulatory and catalytic functions, for example, contain several sites which interact in a highly specific manner such that the affinity of a given site for the substrate is markedly influenced by the state of binding at the other sites. But whereas we know very little of the structure of most enzymes of this type, hemoglobin is one of a very small number of biological molecules whose immensely intricate machinery has been revealed to us. We owe this insight to the group under the leadership of M. F. PERUTZ in Cambridge, England, whose research over a period of several decades culminated in a detailed description of the three-dimensional structure. As a result of this work, there is now a precise structural basis for attempts to formulate a general theoretical framework within which it may be possible to understand the relationship between structure and function as well as the correlation of diverse molecular properties. Hemoglobin has thus assumed the role of a prototype or model system whose study acquires ramifications extending beyond its own function as an oxygen transport system.

Two main topics have been selected from the vast storehouse of accumulated knowledge concerning hemoglobin and its many derivatives: 1. the cooperative characteristics of hemoglobin in the oxygenation process and 2. the quantum mechanical description of iron in the rather special environment existing in hemoglobin. A comprehensive theory would encompass both topics and would be capable of demonstrating the logical connections between them. Unfortunately, we have not yet achieved this level of understanding, though the early stages of a theoretical structure are already discernible and provide grounds for optimism. We must therefore be content with a presentation in which each of the main topics is treated largely independently of the other.

A further objective of the choice of subject matter is to illustrate the manner in which physics—together with chemistry and biology—participates in a multidisciplinary attack on some kinds of biological problems. The chief emphasis in this book is, therefore, on the physical aspects, in the hope that it will make some contribution to a reduction of the barrier between physics and biology and encourage those physicists who have discovered that their methods and concepts often have interesting—sometimes even exciting—applications in the biological realm. In this connection, F. J. Dyson (1970) once remarked that "physics should keep in close touch with biology, as biology rather than physics is likely to be the central ground of scientific advance during the remainder of the century". The history of science has not been especially kind to prognosticators, but there is little doubt that the boundaries between the traditional disciplines are becoming more diffuse as ideas and techniques from one area of science are fruitfully applied in other areas.

I thank Dr. M. F. Perutz for his kind permission to reproduce several figures from his publications and Mrs. H. C. Denney for typing the manuscript and her excellent assistance with the proofs.

Stanford, January 1974   M. Weissbluth

Contents

Chapter I

Amino Acids, Peptides and Proteins

In this chapter we summarize the nomenclature and certain properties pertaining to proteins and their constituents. Additional information is readily available in standard works on biochemistry such as FRUTON and SIMMONDS (1958), EDSALL and WYMAN (1958), MAHLER and CORDES (1967), DICKERSON and GEIS (1969) and LEHNINGER (1970).

1.1 Amino Acids

The general structural formula for an amino acid is shown in Fig. 1.1. The carbon atom to which the amino ($-NH_2$) and carboxyl ($-COOH$) groups are attached is designated as the α-carbon; R is a side chain, i.e. a chemical group which varies from one amino acid to another. The amino group is basic, meaning that under appropriate conditions it can accept a proton and become $-NH_3^+$ (cation); on the other hand the carboxyl group is acidic so that upon donation of a proton it becomes $-COO^-$ (anion). As a consequence, amino acids in aqueous solution may exist as dipolar ions (Fig. 1.2).

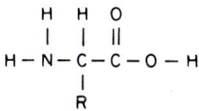

Fig. 1.1. Amino acid in neutral form   Fig. 1.2. Amino acid as a dipolar ion

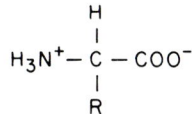

The amino acids that occur in hemoglobin are listed in Table 1.1. Included are the structural formulas (in neutral form), the labeling conventions according to EDSALL *et al.* (1966), the pK_a and pI values, and finally, an indication as to whether the side chains are *polar* or *nonpolar* and if polar, the sign of the net charge at pH 7. The significance of the pK_a and pI values may be illustrated by referring to glycine. For the carboxyl group we have the equilibrium

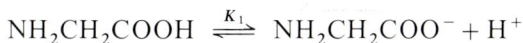

$$NH_2CH_2COOH \xrightarrow{K_1} NH_2CH_2COO^- + H^+$$

Table 1.1. *Structural formulas of amino acids (in neutral form), conventions for labeling of atoms, pK_a and pI values, and classification of side chains into polar and nonpolar groups. When the side chain contains a polar group the sign of the charge at pH 7 is shown in parentheses*

	GLYCINE (GLY)	ALANINE (ALA)	VALINE (VAL)	LEUCINE (LEU)	SERINE (SER)
Structure	H–N–C–C–O–H	H–N–C–C–O–H; H–C–H	H–N–C–C–O–H; H–C–C–H; H–C–H	H–N–C–C–O–H; H–C–H; H–C–C–H; H–C–H	H–N–C–C–O–H; H–C–H; O–H
Labeling	$C_\alpha - C'$	$C_\alpha - C'$; C_β	$C_\alpha - C'$; $C_\beta - C_{\gamma 2}$; $C_{\gamma 1}$	$C_\alpha - C'$; C_β; $C_\gamma - C_{\delta 2}$; $C_{\delta 1}$	$C_\alpha - C'$; C_β; O_γ
pK_a	2.34; 9.6	2.35; 9.69	2.32; 9.62	2.36; 9.60	2.21; 9.15
pI	5.97	6.02	5.97	5.98	5.68
	NONPOLAR	NONPOLAR	NONPOLAR	NONPOLAR	POLAR (0)

	THREONINE (THR)	ASPARTIC ACID (ASP)	GLUTAMIC ACID (GLU)	ASPARAGINE (ASN)	GLUTAMINE (GLN)
Structure	H–N–C–C–O–H; H–C–O–H; H–C–H; H	H–N–C–C–O–H; H–C–H; C=O; O–H	H–N–C–C–O–H; H–C–H; H–C–H; C=O; O–H	H–N–C–C–O–H; H–C–H; C=O; H–N–H	H–N–C–C–O–H; H–C–H; H–C–H; C=O; H–N–H
Labeling	$C_\alpha - C'$; $C_\beta - O_{\gamma 1}$; $C_{\gamma 2}$	$C_\alpha - C'$; C_β; $C_\gamma - O_{\delta 2}$; $O_{\delta 1}$	$C_\alpha - C'$; C_β; C_γ; $C_\delta - O_{\epsilon 2}$; $O_{\epsilon 1}$	$C_\alpha - C'$; C_β; $C_\gamma - O_{\delta 2}$; $N_{\delta 1}$	$C_\alpha - C'$; C_β; C_γ; $C_\delta - O_{\epsilon 2}$; $N_{\epsilon 1}$
pK_2	2.63; 10.43	2.09 – α CARBOXYL; 3.86 – β CARBOXYL; 9.82	2.19 – α CARBOXYL; 4.25 – γ CARBOXYL; 9.67	2.02; 8.8	2.17; 9.13
pI	6.53	2.87	3.22	5.41	5.65
	POLAR (0)	POLAR (−)	POLAR (−)	POLAR (0)	POLAR (0)

Table 1.1. (continued)

	LYSINE (LYS)	HISTIDINE (HIS)	ARGININE (ARG)	PHENYLALANINE(PHE)	TYROSINE (TYR)
	H H O H-N-C-C-O-H H-C-H H-C-H H-C-H H-C-H H-N-H	H H O H-N-C-C-O-H H-C-H C=C-H H-N N C H	H H O H-N-C-C-O-H H-C-H H-C-H H-C-H N-H C=NH H-N-H	H H O H-N-C-C-O-H H-C-H	H H O H-N-C-C-O-H H-C-H O-H
	$C_\alpha - C'$ C_β C_γ C_δ C_ϵ N_ζ	$C_\alpha - C'$ C_β $C_\gamma - C_{\delta 2}$ $N_{\delta 1} \quad N_{\epsilon 2}$ $C_{\epsilon 1}$	$C_\alpha - C'$ C_β C_γ C_δ N_ϵ $C_\zeta - N_{\eta 1}$ $N_{\eta 2}$	$C_\alpha - C'$ C_β C_γ $C_{\delta 2} \quad C_{\delta 1}$ $C_{\epsilon 2} \quad C_{\epsilon 1}$ C_ζ	$C_\alpha - C'$ C_β C_γ $C_{\delta 2} \quad C_{\delta 1}$ $C_{\epsilon 2} \quad C_{\epsilon 1}$ C_ζ O_η
pK_a	2.18 8.95 − α AMINO 10.53 − ε AMINO	1.82 6.0 − IMIDAZOLE 9.17	2.17 9.04 − α AMINO 12.48 − GUANIDINO	1.83 9.13	2.20 9.11 − α AMINO 10.07 − PHENOLIC HYDROXYL
pI	9.74	7.58	10.76	5.98	5.65
	POLAR (+)	POLAR (O)	POLAR (+)	NONPOLAR	POLAR (O)

	TRYPTOPHAN (TRY)	CYSTEINE (CYH)	METHIONINE (MET)	PROLINE (PRO)	
	H H O H-N-C-C-O-H H-C-H C=C H N-H	H H O H-N-C-C-O-H H-C-H S-H	H H O H-N-C-C-O-H H-C-H H-C-H S H-C-H H	H O H-N-C-C-O-H H-C-H H-C-H C H H	
	$C_\alpha - C'$ C_β $C_\gamma - C_{\delta 1}$ $C_{\delta 2} \quad N_\epsilon$ $C_{\epsilon 2} \quad C_{\epsilon 1}$ $C_{\zeta 2} \quad C_{\zeta 1}$ C_η	$C_\alpha - C'$ C_β S_γ	$C_\alpha - C'$ C_β C_γ S_δ C_ϵ	$N - C_\alpha - C'$ $C_\delta \quad C_\beta$ C_γ	
pK_a	2.38 9.39	1.71 8.33 − SULFHYDRYL 10.78 − α AMINO	2.28 9.21	1.99 10.60	
pI	5.88	5.02	5.75	6.10	
	POLAR (O)	POLAR (O)	NONPOLAR	NONPOLAR	

in which $NH_2CH_2COO^-$ is known as the conjugate base and K_1 is related to the equilibrium concentrations by

$$K_1 = \frac{[NH_2CH_2COO^-][H^+]}{[NH_2CH_2COOH]}$$

where the symbol [ ] stands for concentration. By definition, with logarithms to base 10,

$$pK_1 = -\log K_1,$$

$$pH = -\log[H^+]$$

so that

$$pK_1 = pH + \log \frac{[NH_2CH_2COOH]}{[NH_2CH_2COO^-]} .$$

Thus pK_1 is that value of pH at which the acid is half dissociated, or

$$[NH_2CH_2COOH] = [NH_2CH_2COO^-] .$$

For glycine $pK_1 = 2.34$; this means that

$$\text{for } pH \gtrless 2.34, \quad [NH_2CH_2COO^-] \gtrless [NH_2CH_2COOH] .$$

More generally,

$$\text{for } pH \gtrless pK, \quad [\text{base}] \gtrless [\text{acid}] \tag{1.1.1}$$

which also indicates that of two acids, the one with the lower pK is the stronger, i.e. at any given pH, the one with the lower pK is more completely dissociated.

There is also an equilibrium associated with the amino group

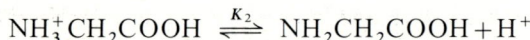

$$NH_3^+CH_2COOH \xrightleftharpoons{K_2} NH_2CH_2COOH + H^+$$

in which $NH_3^+CH_2COOH$ is known as the conjugate acid. Repeating the previous steps

$$pK_2 = pH + \log \frac{[NH_3^+CH_2COOH]}{[NH_2CH_2COOH]} .$$

For glycine $pK_2 = 9.6$ and

$$\text{for } pH \gtrless 9.6, \quad [NH_2CH_2COOH] \gtrless [NH_3^+CH_2COOH]$$

which is again of the same form as the relation (1.1.1).

Similar equilibria and their corresponding pK-values are associated with ionizable groups in the side chains. In aspartic acid, for example, there is an additional carboxyl group in the side chain with a pK of 3.86; lysine has an amino group in the side chain with a pK of 10.53. From Eq. (1.1.1), we deduce that at pH 7 aspartic acid is negatively charged while lysine is positive. In Table 1.1 all pK-values are labeled pK_a to signify that it is the dissociation of the acid or conjugate acid which is being characterized. When no further description is given, the low values of pK_a, 2—4, refer to the α-carboxyl and the high values, 8—10, to the α-amino groups.

Returing to glycine, we note that

$$1/2(pK_1+pK_2)=pH+1/2\log\frac{[NH_3^+CH_2COOH]}{[NH_2CH_2COO^-]}.$$

In the special case when

$$[NH_3^+CH_2COOH]=[NH_2CH_2COO^-],$$
$$pH=1/2(pK_1+pK_2)=pI. \qquad (1.1.2)$$

pI is the isoelectric point i.e. the pH at which the net electric charge is zero. For glycine pI is 5.97 and at this pH the average charge on a glycine molecule is zero. When

$$pH \lesseqgtr 5.97, \quad \text{net charge} = \begin{cases} + \\ 0 \\ - \end{cases}.$$

More generally, when ionizable side chains are present, Eq. (1.1.2) is no longer valid, but we can still define pI as the pH value at which the net electric charge of the amino acid is, on average, zero.

Amino acids—except for glycine—are optically active as a result of the asymmetric α carbon. If we look back from the H atom to the α carbon and find that the other groups are disposed in the clockwise order R, amino, carboxyl, such an amino acid is said to be in the L form. This is the naturally occurring form, although a D form can be obtained by interchanging the positions of two groups attached to the α carbon. The designations L and D are purely formal and do not refer to the rotation of polarized light to the right or left.

As we examine the list of amino acids the following features may be noted:

1. Glycine, alanine, valine and leucine have nonionizable side chains which remain uncharged over a wide range of pH. These amino acids are therefore classified as nonpolar. In aqueous solution nonpolar substances tend to arrange themselves so as to exclude water and thereby force the water molecules in their immediate vicinity to adopt a cage-like structure with a consequent overall reduction in entropy. For this reason, they are also described as *hydrophobic*, to indicate that an expenditure of several kilocalories of free energy is required to transfer a mole of hydrophobic substance from a nonpolar medium to a polar one like water.

2. Serine and threonine contain aliphatic hydroxyl groups in their side chains, which also remain uncharged over a wide range of pH; they are therefore said to be polar but neutral. They also have the potential of forming hydrogen bonds such as $-O-H---N-$.

3. The side chains in aspartic acid and glutamic acid contain carboxyl groups which can be ionized by detachment of a proton. They are therefore classified as polar, acidic (proton donors), and at pH 7 they carry a negative charge; they may also participate in hydrogen-bond formation.

4. Asparagine and glutamine are related to aspartic acid and glutamic acid respectively. The OH group in the acid is replaced by NH_2, which remains uncharged over a wide range of pH; they are therefore polar but neutral.

5. Lysine, histidine and arginine are classified as polar, basic amino acids because the side chains are proton acceptors. Thus in lysine there is an amino group, while histidine and arginine contain imidazole and guanidinium groups respectively, as shown in Figs. 1.3 and 1.4, at pH 7; lysine and arginine are positively charged but histidine only to a slight extent.

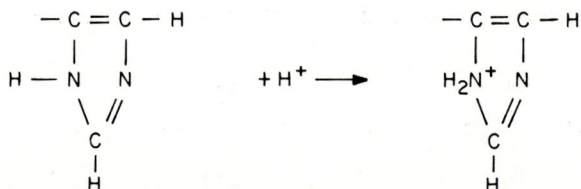

Fig. 1.3. Imidazole group of histidine in neutral and ionized form

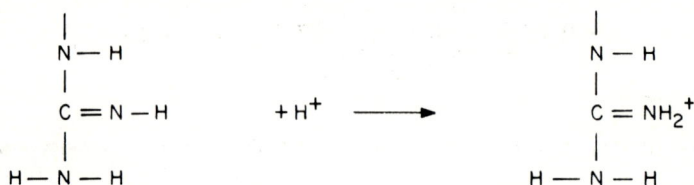

Fig. 1.4. Guanidinium group of arginine in neutral and ionized form

6. Phenylalanine, tryptophan and tyrosine contain aromatic groups in their side chains, which confer upon them the ability to absorb light in the ultraviolet region, in the vicinity of 2800 Å. Phenylalanine is nonpolar, tryptophan and tyrosine are both polar but neutral at pH 7.

7. Cysteine and methionine are characterized by the presence of reactive sulfur in the side chains. The former is polar and neutral and the latter is nonpolar.

8. Proline has an α-imino group (NH) in place of an α-amino (NH$_2$) group; it is nonpolar.

1.2 Peptides

Two amino acids may join to form a *dipeptide* by eliminating a water molecule between the —COOH of one and the —NH$_2$ of the other. This process is illustrated in Fig. 1.5, with the *peptide* unit defined as the group —C—CO—NH—C— shown inside the dashed area. Referring to Fig. 1.6, which shows the structural details of the peptide unit, we note that the C_{α}—C' bond length is 1.53 Å and the C_{α}—N distance is 1.47 Å. Both these values are typical of single bonds, so that free rotation about these bonds may be expected. On the other hand, the C'—N bond in the peptide linkage is only 1.32 Å long, which is a good indication of at least partial double-bond character. The consequences of this are, first of all, to hinder the rotation about the C'—N bond—the barrier to rotation is

about 21 kcal/mole—and secondly to force the peptide unit into a planar configuration.

Since the two ends of the dipeptide are —COOH and —NH$_2$, as in a single
amino acid, the process described above may continue to the formation of long
chains known as *polypeptides*. A schematic representation of a polypeptide chain
consisting of four amino-acid *residues* is shown in Fig. 1.7, where the term residue
refers to the group of atoms —NH—CHR—CO—. It is customary to refer to
the amino and carboxyl ends of a chain as the N and C terminals respectively.

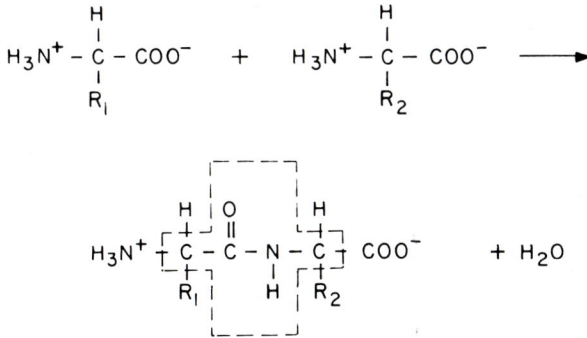

Fig. 1.5. Formation of a dipeptide. The group of atoms inside the dashed enclosure is the peptide unit

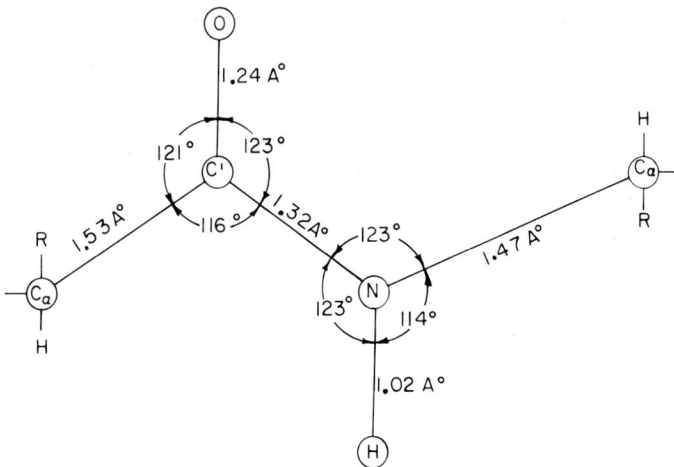

Fig. 1.6. Bond distances and angles of the peptide unit

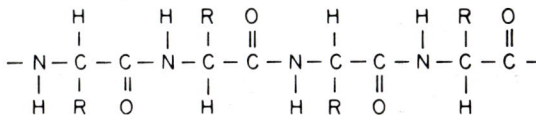

Fig. 1.7. A portion of a polypeptide chain consisting of 4 residues: each residue is a group
—NH—CHR—CO—

1.3 Proteins

The basic structural elements of proteins are polypeptide chains; some proteins—hemoglobin among them—contain additional groups which will be described later. It is customary to subdivide protein structures into primary through quaternary; these will now be defined.

Primary structure refers to the number and sequence of amino acids in the polypeptide chains.

The spatial configuration of the polypeptide chain is the secondary structure. In the first instance there may be no special configuration, in which case the chain is said to exist as a random coil such as is illustrated schematically in Fig. 1.8. A second important configuration is the α helix (PAULING et al., 1951) shown in Fig. 1.9. In this structure the planar peptide groups arrange themselves into a helix with 3.6 residues per turn; the distance between successive turns (pitch) is 5.4 Å and the radius of the helix, measured to the α carbons, is 2.3 Å. An important feature of the α helix is that there are hydrogen bonds between an α imino nitrogen (NH) in one residue and an α carboxyl oxygen (CO) three residues further along the chain; the hydrogen bonds are approximately parallel to the axis of the helix. In another notation, the α helix is said to be a 3.6_{13} helix, meaning that there are 3.6 turns per residue and 13 atoms within a loop containing one hydrogen bond. Other helical arrangements, e.g. the 3_{10} helix, are possible but less common. Whether a polypeptide exists as a random coil or in a helical form depends on external conditions such as the nature of the solvent; thus, solvents which disrupt the hydrogen bonds in the helix will cause the polypeptide to assume a randomly coiled form. Secondary structures may contain sections of both random coil and helical configurations, and when the latter occur in natural proteins, they are right-handed helices of L amino acids. Still another configuration is the β form in which amino-acid chains have an extended zig-zag form. Such chains are usually held together in sheets; they are not present in hemoglobin.

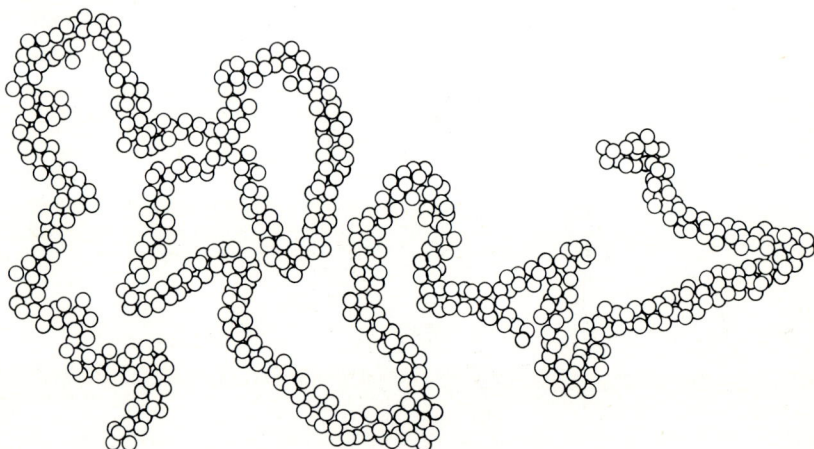

Fig. 1.8. Model of a protein in the configuration of a random coil

The helical and nonhelical sections of a polypeptide chain may assume complicated three-dimensional shapes which are stabilized by a variety of interactions among the side chains e.g. ionic bonds, hydrogen bonds, van-der-Waals
forces etc. This is the tertiary structure. Of significance here are the hydrophobic
interactions; these manifest themselves in the tendency of the chain to fold into
a configuration such that the nonpolar side chains are largely removed from the
aqueous medium and transferred to the interior. Finally, several polypeptide
chains may fold into one another to form a still more complicated three-dimensional structure which is then known as the quaternary structure.

We have seen that some amino acids contain ionizable side chains. Proteins
in solution, therefore, generally carry a net charge whose sign and magnitude
depend on the pH; this property classifies them as polyelectrolytes. An important
consequence is that proteins will migrate in an electric field. As the pH is varied
from strongly acidic (low pH) to strongly alkaline (high pH), the charge on a
protein will vary from a large positive to a large negative value. At some intermediate pH, the net charge will be zero—this is the isoelectric point—and the
protein will not migrate in an electric field.

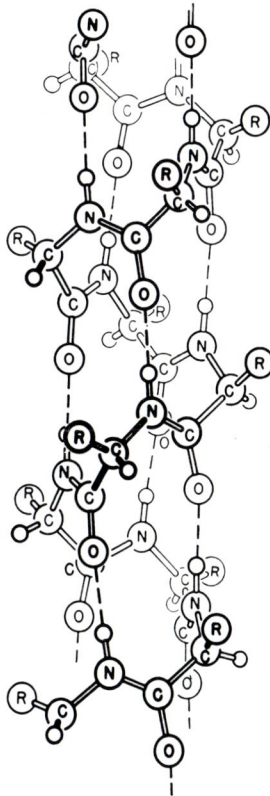

Fig. 1.9. A right-handed α helix consisting of L-amino acid residues

Chapter II

Hemoglobin

2.1 Primary Structure

The hemoglobin molecule is composed of four subunits, each of which contains a polypeptide chain. The chains are of two types—designated α and β—which differ primarily in the number and sequence of amino-acid residues. For horse hemoglobin (PERUTZ, 1969a), the sequences are shown in Table 2.1; an α chain contains 141 and a β chain 146 residues, making a total of 574 residues for the whole molecule. Each residue is labeled in two ways: by its position in the chain, counting from the amino end (N terminal) and by its position in an identifiable portion of the tertiary structure (see section 2.4).

In the α chain, the 87th residue is histidine F 8 (87α) and in the β chain there is a histidine in position F 8 (92β). A heme group, illustrated in Fig. 2.1, is attached to each of the four histidines. The heme consists of an iron atom (Fe^{2+} or Fe^{3+}) attached to a planar organic structure belonging to a class

Table 2.1. *The sequence of amino acid residues in the α and β chains of horse hemoglobin, numbered from the amino ends and labeled with reference to the helical and nonhelical sections of the chain* (PERUTZ 1969a)

		α			β					α			β	
1	VAL	NA	2	VAL	NA	1		21	ALA	B	2	GLU	B	3
2	LEU		3	GLN		2		22	GLY		3	GLU		4
3	SER	A	1	LEU		3		23	GLU		4	VAL		5
4	ALA		2	SER	A	1		24	TYR		5	GLY		6
5	ALA		3	GLY		2		25	GLY		6	GLY		7
6	ASP		4	GLU		3		26	ALA		7	GLU		8
7	LYS		5	GLU		4		27	GLU		8	ALA		9
8	THR		6	LYS		5		28	ALA		9	LEU		10
9	ASN		7	ALA		6		29	LEU		10	GLY		11
10	VAL		8	ALA		7		30	GLU		11	ARG		12
11	LYS		9	VAL		8		31	ARG		12	LEU		13
12	ALA		10	LEU		9		32	MET		13	LEU		14
13	ALA		11	ALA		10		33	PHE		14	VAL		15
14	TRY		12	LEU		11		34	LEU		15	VAL		16
15	SER		13	TRY		12		35	GLY		16	TYR	C	1
16	LYS		14	ASP		13		36	PHE	C	1	PRO		2
17	VAL		15	LYS		14		37	PRO		2	TRY		3
18	GLY		16	VAL		15		38	THR		3	THR		4
19	GLY	AB	1	ASN	B	1		39	THR		4	GLN		5
20	HIS	B	1	GLU		2		40	LYS		5	ARG		6

Table 2.1. (continued)

	α			β				α			β		
41	THR	C	6	PHE	C	7	94	ASP	G	1	ASP	FG	1
42	TYR		7	PHE	CD	1	95	PRO		2	LYS		2
43	PHE	CD	1	ASP		2	96	VAL		3	LEU		3
44	PRO		2	SER		3	97	ASN		4	HIS		4
45	HIS		3	PHE		4	98	PHE		5	VAL		5
46	PHE		4	GLY		5	99	LYS		6	ASP	G	1
47	ASP		5	ASP		6	100	LEU		7	PRO		2
48	LEU		7	LEU		7	101	LEU		8	GLU		3
49	SER		8	SER		8	102	SER		9	ASN		4
50	HIS	D	6	ASP	D	1	103	HIS		10	PHE		5
51	GLY		7	PRO		2	104	CYH		11	ARG		6
52	SER	E	1	GLY		3	105	LEU		12	LEU		7
53	ALA		2	ALA		4	106	LEU		13	LEU		8
54	GLN		3	VAL		5	107	SER		14	GLY		9
55	VAL		4	MET		6	108	THR		15	ASN		10
56	LYS		5	GLY		7	109	LEU		16	VAL		11
57	ALA		6	ASN	E	1	110	ALA		17	LEU		12
58	HIS		7	PRO		2	111	VAL		18	ALA		13
59	GLY		8	LYS		3	112	HIS		19	LEU		14
60	LYS		9	VAL		4	113	LEU	GH	1	VAL		15
61	LYS		10	LYS		5	114	PRO		2	VAL		16
62	VAL		11	ALA		6	115	ASN		3	ALA		17
63	ALA		12	HIS		7	116	ASP		4	ARG		18
64	ASP		13	GLY		8	117	PHE		5	HIS		19
65	GLY		14	LYS		9	118	THR	H	1	PHE	GH	1
66	LEU		15	LYS		10	119	PRO		2	GLY		2
67	THR		16	VAL		11	120	ALA		3	LYS		3
68	LEU		17	LEU		12	121	VAL		4	ASP		4
69	ALA		18	HIS		13	122	HIS		5	PHE		5
70	VAL		19	SER		14	123	ALA		6	THR	H	1
71	GLY		20	PHE		15	124	SER		7	PRO		2
72	HIS	EF	1	GLY		16	125	LEU		8	GLU		3
73	LEU		2	GLU		17	126	ASP		9	LEU		4
74	ASP		3	GLY		18	127	LYS		10	GLN		5
75	ASP		4	VAL		19	128	PHE		11	ALA		6
76	LEU		5	HIS		20	129	LEU		12	SER		7
77	PRO		6	HIS	EF	1	130	SER		13	TYR		8
78	GLY		7	LEU		2	131	SER		14	GLN		9
79	ALA		8	ASP		3	132	VAL		15	LYS		10
80	LEU	F	1	ASN		4	133	SER		16	VAL		11
81	SER		2	LEU		5	134	THR		17	VAL		12
82	ASP		3	LYS		6	135	VAL		18	ALA		13
83	LEU		4	GLY		7	136	LEU		19	GLY		14
84	SER		5	THR		8	137	THR		20	VAL		15
85	ASN		6	PHE	F	1	138	SER		21	ALA		16
86	LEU		7	ALA		2	139	LYS	HC	1	ASN		17
87	HIS		8	ALA		3	140	TYR		2	ALA		18
88	ALA		9	LEU		4	141	ARG		3	LEU		19
89	HIS	FG	1	SER		5	142				ALA		20
90	LYS		2	GLU		6	143				HIS		21
91	LEU		3	LEU		7	144				LYS	HC	1
92	ARG		4	HIS		8	145				TYR		2
93	VAL		5	CYH		9	146				HIS		3

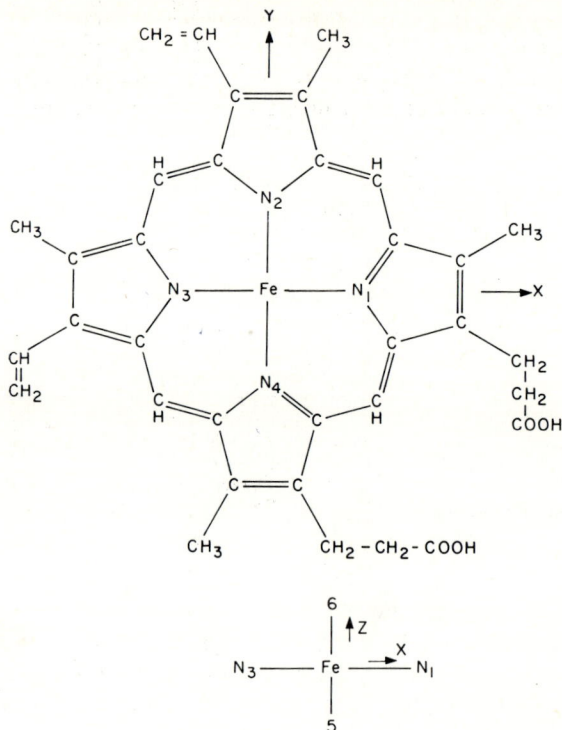

Fig. 2.1. The heme complex and its coordinate system

of compounds known as porphyrins. These contain four 5-membered ring structures (pyrroles) with interconnections (methine bridges) and side chains attached to the pyrroles. The particular porphyrin found in hemoglobin is protoporphyrin IX, which is distinguished from other porphyrins by the side chains— four methyls ($-CH_3$), two vinyls ($-C=CH_2$) and two propionic acids ($-CH_2-CH_2-COOH$). In the plane of the heme the iron atom is attached (liganded) to the four pyrrole nitrogens; in a direction perpendicular to the heme plane there is an attachment (labeled 5) by means of a covalent bond between iron an nitrogen $N_{\varepsilon 2}$ on the imidazole of histidine F8 (Fig. 2.2). This residue is therefore known as the proximal or heme-linked histidine. Another attachment position is available in the opposite direction, also perpendicular to the heme plane; this is position 6, to which various atoms or molecules, including O_2, may be bound. The out-of-plane atoms or molecules that occupy positions 5 and 6 are the axial ligands; a few examples of groups that can occupy position 6 are listed in Table 2.2.

Thus, hemoglobin is a tetramer consisting of four subunits ($\alpha_1 \alpha_2 \beta_1 \beta_2$); each subunit is a combination of a polypeptide chain, which is the protein or globin part of hemoglobin, and a heme. The latter is the functional unit or active site to which a molecule of oxygen (or some other ligand) may be bound. The total molecular weight is about 67000; there are some 10000 atoms, 4 of which are iron; the others are C, H, O, N, S. Hemoglobins from different species have different amino-acid sequences; indeed, only seven locations are invariably occupied by the same residues, and these sites are mainly around the heme and in contacts between subunits. Even within a single species there are numerous variations.

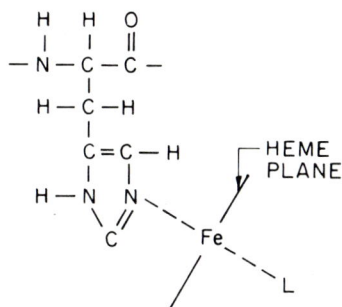

Fig. 2.2. Attachment of heme iron to $N_{\varepsilon 2}$ of histidine F 8. L represents a ligand in the sixth position

Among humans, for example, there are over 100 mutant varieties which differ from normal adult hemoglobin (HbA) in having some residues in either α or β chains replaced by others. The effect of a replacement of this kind on the physiological function of the molecule depends on the location of the residue; the most sensitive regions are near the hemes and in the contact regions between unlike chains.

A molecule closely related to hemoglobin is myoglobin which is found in muscle; in contrast to the oxygen-transport characteristics of hemoglobin, myoglobin functions as an oxygen-storage system. It consists of a single chain of amino-acid residues and contains one heme to which an oxygen molecule, or

Table 2.2. *Some derivatives of hemoglobin and their spins. Note that each molecule of hemoglobin binds 4 ligands; thus, for example,* HbO_2 *is an abbreviated version of* $Hb(O_2)_4$. *The same nomenclature applies to the other derivatives*

	Ligand in Sixth Position	Spin
Ferrous Derivatives		
Oxyhemoglobin (HbO_2)	O_2	0
Carboxyhemoglobin (HbCO)	CO	0
Deoxyhemoglobin (Hb)	None	2
NO-hemoglobin (NbNO)	NO	0
Ferric Derivatives		
Acid methemoglobin (HbH_2O)	H_2O	5/2
(methemoglobin, ferrihemoglobin)		
Alkaline methemoglobin (HbOH)	OH^-	1/2, 5/2
(ferrihemoglobin hydroxide)		
Ferrihemoglobin fluoride (HbF)	F^-	5/2
Ferrihemoglobin azide (HbN_3)	N_3^-	1/2
Ferrihemoglobin cyanide (HbCN)	CN^-	1/2
(cyanomethemoglobin)		

some other ligand, may be bound. The molecular weight is 18 000; myoglobin may therefore be loosely regarded as similar to one subunit of hemoglobin.

Hemoglobin with oxygen bound to each heme (in the sixth position) is known as oxyhemoglobin; when the sixth position is vacant, the molecule is called deoxyhemoglobin. In both cases the heme is said to be reduced, meaning that the iron is in the ferrous state (Fe^{2+}). This is the traditional description. However, there appears to be evidence, both theoretical and experimental, to suggest that there is a considerable transfer of electronic charge from the iron to the oxygen in oxyhemoglobin. We shall go into these matters in later chapters, but at this stage our purpose is to remark that from a physical standpoint, the distinction between the ferrous (Fe^{2+}) and ferric (Fe^{3+}) state in oxyhemoglobin is rather blurred. Nevertheless, for purposes of nomenclature, as in Table 2.2 we follow tradition and refer to oxyhemoglobin as a ferrous compound.

As mentioned above, atoms or molecules other than O_2 may occupy the sixth position. These are called derivatives of hemoglobin. When the heme is oxidized, i.e. the iron atom is in the ferric (Fe^{3+}) state, the derivative is usually known as ferrihemoglobin, although some special names have come into usage (Table 2.2). Derivatives in which the heme is reduced are sometimes called ferro-hemoglobin. Hemoglobin is also used as a generic name when reference to the oxidation state is of no consequence. Liganded hemoglobin is a general name for any derivative with a ligand (i.e. atom or molecule) occupying the sixth position; this includes all hemoglobin derivatives except, of course, deoxyhemoglobin.

A somewhat confusing convention which remains in vogue is to write HbO_2 for oxyhemoglobin. Since oxyhemoglobin actually binds 4 oxygen molecules, a more rigorous designation would be $Hb(O_2)_4$. It is also customary to shorten the notation for other derivatives; thus HbCO is written for $Hb(CO)_4$, HbCN for $Hb(CN)_4$, etc.

In this book we focus attention on mammalian oxy- and deoxyhemoglobin and the processes involved in the transition from one to the other. Nevertheless, experiments with other derivatives have contributed to our understanding of the oxygenation process; it would therefore be improper to ignore them. A description of structure or properties, without further identification of the derivative, refers to oxy- or deoxyhemoglobin.

2.2 Spin States

It is often useful to characterize hemoglobin derivatives according to the spin state of the iron atom. Though this subject is treated in Chapter V, a brief introduction is pertinent at this stage.

A neutral iron atom has 26 electrons, 18 of which reside in closed shells ($1s^2 2s^2 2p^6 3s^2 3p^6$) while the remaining 8 have the orbital configuration $(3d)^6(4s)^2$. In hemoglobin, as we have seen, iron is in either the ferric (Fe^{3+}) or the ferrous (Fe^{2+}) state; in the former case the orbital configuration outside closed shells is $(3d)^5$ and in the latter it is $(3d)^6$. The $3d$ shell consists of five orbitals which can accomodate a maximum of 10 electrons provided their spins are paired (anti-parallel) as required by the exclusion principle. When there are fewer than 10 electrons, various arrangements are possible. Specifically, with 5 electrons there may be one electron in each d orbital; the spins may all be aligned parallel to one another resulting in a total spin $S = 5/2$ as shown in Fig. 2.3 a. Other possible arrangements are shown in Figs. 2.3 b and 2.3 c and lead to $S = 3/2$ and $1/2$. With 6 electrons, similar arrangements lead to $S = 2, 1, 0$, as shown in Fig. 2.3 d, e and f

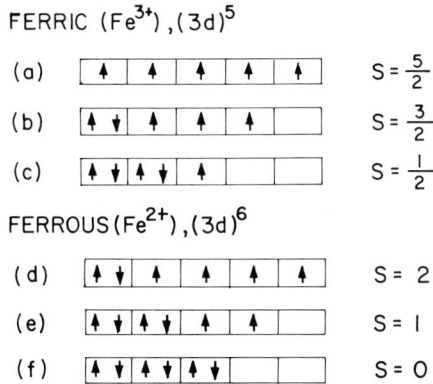

FERRIC $(Fe^{3+}), (3d)^5$

(a) $S = \dfrac{5}{2}$

(b) $S = \dfrac{3}{2}$

(c) $S = \dfrac{1}{2}$

FERROUS $(Fe^{2+}), (3d)^6$

(d) $S = 2$

(e) $S = 1$

(f) $S = 0$

Fig. 2.3. Spin alignments of $3d$ electrons in Fe^{3+} and Fe^{2+}

None of the various derivatives of hemoglobin has intermediate spin values. Thus, ferric derivatives exist with $S = 0$ or 2 but not 1 while the ferric types have $S = 1/2$ or $5/2$ but not $3/2$. The spins of some of the common derivatives are given in Table 2.2. Deoxyhemoglobin is unique in that the sixth position is vacant, so that the iron is 5-coordinated; it is the only ferrous derivative with high spin $(S = 2)$, and it is therefore paramagnetic. All other ferrous derivatives are 6-coordinated, have low spin $(S = 0)$ and are therefore diamagnetic. The ferric derivatives are all 6-coordinated, have nonvanishing spins $(S = 1/2$ or $5/2)$ and are therefore paramagnetic. It must be remembered, however, that the globin or protein part of hemoglobin is diamagnetic.

The stable isotopes of iron have mass numbers 54, 56, 57, and 58, with relative abundances of 5.84, 91.68, 2.17 and 0.31 % respectively. Only ^{57}Fe has a non-vanishing nuclear spin $(1/2)$ and a magnetic moment $(<0.05$ nuclear magnetons). There is therefore no quadrupole interaction with the nucleus in the ground state, and the contribution of the magnetic hyperfine interaction to electron spin resonance is negligible. Nevertheless, the presence of ^{57}Fe, despite its low abundance, makes it possible to observe Mossbauer resonance in natural (i.e. isotopically unenriched) hemoglobin.

2.3 Heme

The structure of the heme has been shown in Fig. 2.1; PERUTZ et al. (1968 b) give complete sets of coordinates for α and β chains, including the heme groups in horse oxyhemoglobin. The origin of the coordinate system is located at the

Table 2.3. *Coordinates of atoms in heme referred to axes shown in Fig. 2.1. The pyrrole carbons are labeled in counterclockwise sequence starting from the pyrrole nitrogen* (PERUTZ *et al.*, 1968 b)

Pyrrole Ring	Atom	Location	Coordinates (Å)		
			x	y	z
	Fe		0.00	0.00	0.00
	C	Methine	2.41	−2.41	0.00
1	C_1	Pyrrole	2.83	−1.10	0.00
1	C_2	Pyrrole	4.22	−0.66	0.00
1	C_A	Prop. Acid	5.45	−1.55	0.00
1	C_B	Prop. Acid	5.83	−1.81	−1.43
1	C_G	Prop. Acid	7.11	−2.66	−1.43
1	O_1	Prop. Acid	7.03	−3.88	−1.43
1	O_2	Prop. Acid	8.17	−2.15	−1.43
1	C_3	Pyrrole	4.22	0.66	0.00
1	C_M	Methyl	5.45	1.55	0.00
1	C_4	Pyrrole	2.83	1.10	0.00
1	N	Pyrrole	2.00	0.00	0.00
	C	Methine	2.41	2.41	0.00
2	C_1	Pyrrole	1.10	2.83	0.00
2	C_2	Pyrrole	0.66	4.22	0.00
2	C_M	Methyl	1.55	5.45	0.00
2	C_3	Pyrrole	−0.66	4.22	0.00
2	C_A	Vinyl	−1.55	5.45	0.00
2	C_B	Vinyl	−1.92	6.01	1.15
2	C_4	Pyrrole	−1.10	2.83	0.00
2	N	Pyrrole	0.00	2.00	0.00
	C	Methine	−2.41	2.41	0.00
3	C_1	Pyrrole	−2.83	1.10	0.00
3	C_2	Pyrrole	−4.22	0.66	0.00
3	C_M	Methyl	−5.45	1.55	0.00
3	C_3	Pyrrole	−4.22	−0.66	0.00
3	C_A	Vinyl	−5.45	−1.55	0.00
3	C_B	Vinyl	−6.01	−1.92	1.15
3	C_4	Pyrrole	−2.83	−1.10	0.00
3	N	Pyrrole	−2.00	0.00	0.00
	C	Methine	−2.41	−2.41	0.00
4	C_1	Pyrrole	−1.10	−2.83	0.00
4	C_2	Pyrrole	−0.66	−4.22	0.00
4	C_M	Methyl	−1.55	−5.45	0.00
4	C_3	Pyrrole	0.66	−4.22	0.00
4	C_A	Prop. Acid	1.55	−5.45	0.00
4	C_B	Prop. Acid	1.81	−5.83	1.43
4	C_G	Prop. Acid	2.66	−7.11	1.43
4	O_1	Prop. Acid	2.15	−8.17	1.43
4	O_2	Prop. Acid	3.88	−7.03	1.43
4	C_4	Pyrrole	1.10	−2.83	0.00
4	N	Pyrrole	0.00	−2.00	0.00

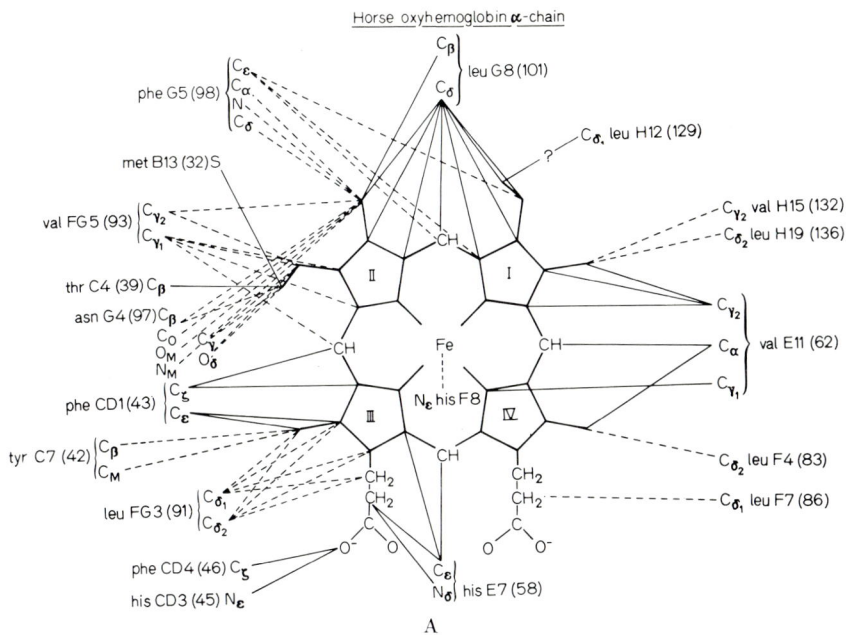

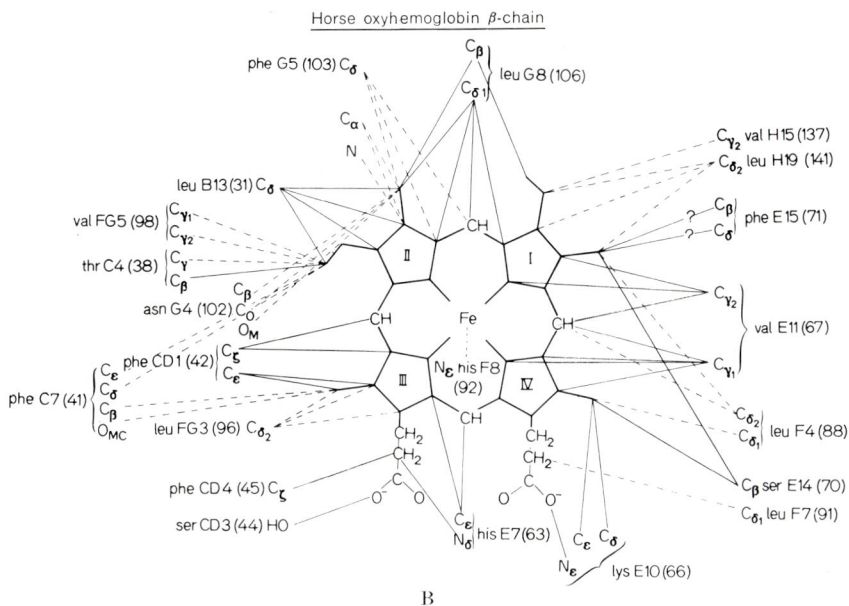

Fig. 2.4 A and B. Contacts between heme and globin in oxyhemoglobin (PERUTZ *et al.*, 1968 b). A α chain, B β chain. All contacts are within 4 A

center of mass of the four heme groups in horse oxyhemoglobin. Table 2.3 lists
the atomic coordinates of heme referred to an origin at the center of the porphyrin
ring and with the axes oriented as in Fig. 2.1.

   Each heme is embedded in a pocket formed by the polypeptide chain to which
it is attached, and the four pockets, each containing a heme, are situated close
to the surface of the molecule. In addition to the covalent bond between iron
and histidine there are van-der-Waals contacts between atoms on the porphyrin
ring and about 60 atoms of the polypeptide chain (Fig. 2.4). Significantly, the
residues in this region are mainly nonpolar. When there is a ligand in the sixth
position it lies in the region bordered by the iron atom, histidine E 7 ($58\,\alpha$ or $63\,\beta$)
and valine E 11 ($62\,\alpha$ or $67\,\beta$).

   Comparison of hemes in oxy- and deoxyhemoglobin reveals that in oxyhemoglobin (as in carboxyhemoglobin) the iron atom is situated in the plane
of the porphyrin ring, the spin $S=0$, and the proximal (heme-linked) nitrogen
$N_{\varepsilon 2}$ of histidine F 8 is approximately $2.0\,\text{Å}$ from the porphyrin plane. Oxygen is
also hydrogen-bonded to histidine E 7 ($58\,\alpha$ or $63\,\beta$). In deoxyhemoglobin, the
iron atom is displaced from the porphyrin plane by about $0.75\,\text{Å}$ in the direction
of the proximal histidine F 8 and the spin $S=2$. The distance between nitrogen
$N_{\varepsilon 2}$ of histidine F 8 and the porphyrin plane also increases to $2.9\,\text{Å}$, resulting in
a slight lengthening of the Fe—$N_{\varepsilon 2}$ bond by $\sim 0.15\,\text{Å}$ (HOARD, 1968, 1971).
Hemes in α and β chains behave in the same fashion. The changes in the heme
structure and the spin state which occur whenever oxygen is bound or released
turn out to be of fundamental importance insofar as the mode of action is concerned; we shall return to this subject in Chapter IV.

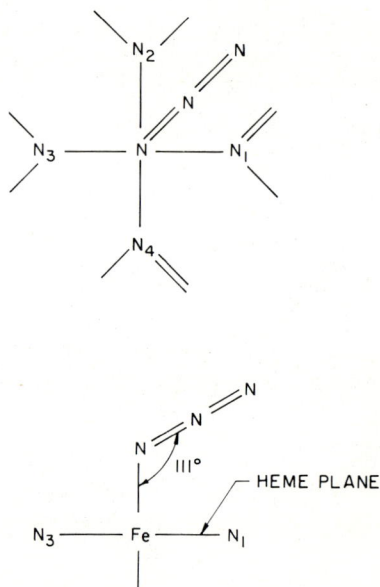

Fig. 2.5. Position of azide in ferrihemoglobin azide (STRYER et al., 1964)

In low-spin ferric derivatives, the iron atom lies close (within 0.05 Å) to the porphyrin plane. In this respect there is a close resemblance to oxyhemoglobin. But in acid methemoglobin, and very likely in other high-spin ferric derivatives, the iron atom is displaced toward the proximal histidine by about 0.3 Å.

The orientation of the oxygen molecule relative to the porphyrin plane is of some interest but is not precisely known. The crystallographic data suggest that the orientation of O_2 is similar to that of N_3^- in myoglobin, which has been determined by STRYER et al. (1964) and is shown in Fig. 2.5 (however, in this connection, see Chapter X).

2.4 Secondary and Tertiary Structure

Essentially all existing knowledge of the three-dimensional structure of hemoglobin has been obtained by PERUTZ and his colleagues by means of X-ray diffraction methods. This work was begun in 1937 and has been under constant improvement and refinement since. We list several of the more recent references: MUIREAD et al. (1967); PERUTZ et al. (1968 a and b); PERUTZ (1969 a and b); MUIRHEAD and GREER (1970); BOLTON and PERUTZ (1970). The history of this subject (PERUTZ, 1964) is indeed remarkable, for it must be remembered that none of the present-day computational facilities existed when the work was started, and even now the structures of only a very small number of biological macromolecules are known in comparable detail.

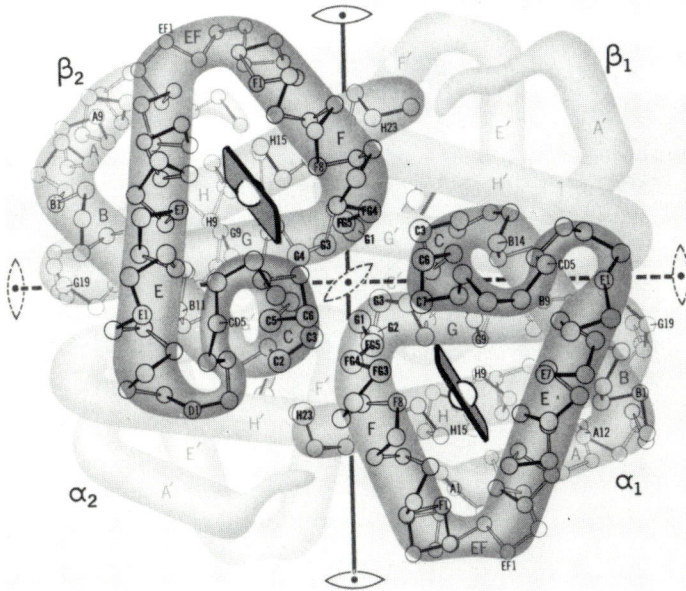

Fig. 2.6. The four chains of oxyhemoglobin (from R. E. DICKERSON and I. GEIS, *The Structure and Action of Proteins*, W. A. Benjamin Co., Menlo Park. Copyright 1969 Dickerson and Geis)

The general shape of a globin chain is illustrated in Fig. 2.6; it consists of helical sections labeled A through H, separated by extended or nonhelical regions labeled according to the helices at either end. Thus CD is a nonhelical section between helices C and D. Except for the short C section, which is a 3_{10} helix, all the other helices are α helices. The residues listed in Table 2.1 are labeled with reference to these sections and are numbered from the N-terminal end of each section. Most of the chain—about 75%—is helical, and the whole chain is folded into a complicated but highly specific three-dimensional pattern which is approximately spherical. The same general description applies to both α chains and β chains, oxygenated or not, of any mammalian hemoglobin; it also applies to myoglobin. However, completion of the high-resolution work at 2.8 Å, first on horse oxyhemoglobin (PERUTZ et al., 1968 a, b) and later on horse deoxy-hemoglobin (BOLTON and PERUTZ, 1970) provided a more detailed description of the three-dimensional shapes and it was then that certain important distinctions between α and β chains were revealed. In the first place, α and β chains do not have identical tertiary structures (conformations)[1], and secondly, each type of chain can exist in one of two possible conformations. These will be labeled r and t. Thus, $^rα, ^tα, ^rβ, ^tβ$ are the possible tertiary conformations of α and β chains. It was also found that when a chain is oxygenated, it is in the r conformation; upon deoxygenation it acquires the t conformation. A unique correlation therefore exists between oxygenation and tertiary conformation. Alternatively, we may regard the affinity for oxygen in the r and t conformations as very high and very low respectively. This is summarized as follows:

r conformation—oxygenated—6-coordinated—low spin $(S=0)$,
t conformation—unliganded—5-coordinated—high spin $(S=2)$.

If, instead of oxygen, other ligands are bound to the heme, again, the chain resides in the r conformation, although in the case of ferric derivatives the spin is not necessarily low. Thus it appears that whenever any kind of ligand is bound to the heme (in the sixth position), the chain resides in the r conformation.

The tertiary structures of the α and β chains are described in great detail in the references cited at the beginning of this section. Insofar as the relationship between structure and function is concerned, the following features appear to be important:

1. The heme pocket in $^tβ$ is restricted and there is no room for a ligand unless the distance between porphyrin and helix E is increased and valine E 11 is moved relative to the porphyrin ring. On the other hand, the same region in $^tα$ is sufficiently large to accommodate a ligand without undergoing distortions.

2. In α chains the C-terminal residue is arginine HC 3 (141 α) and next to it is tyrosine HC 2 (140 α), which, in deoxyhemoglobin, sits in a pocket formed by sections of helix F and helix H. In oxyhemoglobin, helix F moves toward helix H

---

[1] In our terminology, structure and conformation are used interchangeably. A structural or conformational change implies a change in the average positions of the atoms brought about, for example, by rotation about bonds. None of the covalent bonds is broken, nor are any new ones formed; however changes may occur in other linkages, such as hydrogen bonds, van-der-Waals interactions or salt bridges.

and constricts the pocket, thereby cansing expulsion of the tyrosine. As a consequence, the C-terminal arginine is displaced.

3. In β chains the C-terminal residue is histidine HC 3 (146 β), and next to it is tyrosine HC 2 (145 β). Here, too, the tyrosine sits in a pocket formed by helices F and H in deoxyhemoglobin, and is forced out of the pocket when the subunit becomes oxygenated. The net result in this case too is displacement of the C-terminal histidine.

2.5 Quaternary Structure

The quaternary structure of hemoglobin is the arrangement of the two α and two β chains relative to one another. It is a highly organized and complex system which precludes any short simple description but, as was stated earlier, the structure is known in detail and the coordinates of every atom are available. We shall now summarize some of the important features.

1. Hemoglobin is approximately spherical in shape with dimensions of $65 \times 55 \times 50$ Å. The four hemes may be said to define an irregular tetrahedron.

2. The quaternary structures appear to be similar for all mammalian hemoglobins.

3. The iron atoms are separated by distances ranging from 25 to 40 Å (Table 2.4).

Table 2.4. *Distances between iron atoms* (Å) (PERUTZ, 1969 a)

	Deoxyhemoglobin	Oxyhemoglobin
$Fe\beta_1 - Fe\beta_2$	39.9	33.4
$Fe\alpha_1 - Fe\alpha_2$	34.9	36.0
$Fe\beta_1 - Fe\alpha_2$ $\}$ $Fe\beta_2 - Fe\alpha_1$	24.7	25.0
$Fe\alpha_1 - Fe\beta_1$ $\}$ $Fe\alpha_2 - Fe\beta_2$	36.9	35.0

4. The four subunits comprising the quaternary structure are held together mainly by nonpolar interactions and a lesser number of salt bridges (electrostatic interactions) and hydrogen bonds. There are no covalent bonds between subunits.

5. There are two quaternary structures or conformations, designated R and T. The conformation of fully oxygenated hemoglobin would be represented by $[{}^r\alpha_1 {}^r\alpha_2 {}^r\beta_1 {}^r\beta_2]^R$. This means that the four subunits, each in the tertiary r conformation, are organized into the quaternary R conformation. Similarly, the conformation of completely deoxygenated hemoglobin would be $[{}^t\alpha_1 {}^t\alpha_2 {}^t\beta_1 {}^t\beta_2]^T$. Other combinations of tertiary and quaternary conformations are possible, at least in principle, though not equally probable, e. g. $[{}^r\alpha_1 {}^r\alpha_2 {}^r\beta_1 {}^r\beta_2]^T$, $[{}^r\alpha_1 {}^r\alpha_2 {}^r\beta_1 {}^r\beta_2]^R$, $[{}^t\alpha_1 {}^t\alpha_2 {}^r\beta_1 {}^r\beta_2]^R$, $[{}^t\alpha_1 {}^t\alpha_2 {}^t\beta_1 {}^t\beta_2]^R$, etc.

6. With certain exceptions, the general tendency is for nonpolar residues to reside in the interior of the molecule or in the regions of contact between subunits; polar residues tend to lie on the surface in contact with the solvent, although a few nonpolar residues are also found on the surface.

7. The hemoglobin molecule has a two-fold symmetry. This means that there is an axis such that one $\alpha\beta$ pair can be superimposed on the other by rotation of 180° about that axis.

The contact regions between chains have received a great deal of attention, since the interactions among subunits must involve such regions in one way or another. These contact regions are customarily defined by the residues from each chain which come close enough to have atoms lying within 4 Å from one another.

With two α and two β chains there are contacts between both like and unlike chains. Contacts between like chains, i.e. $\alpha_1\alpha_2$ and $\beta_1\beta_2$, are rather tenuous and those that do exist are mainly salt bridges and hydrogen bonds. Contacts between unlike chains are much more extensive; apart from a few hydrogen bonds, these contacts are mainly between nonpolar residues. As a consequence of the hydrophobic effect, the transfer of one of these residues from the nonpolar environment of the contact to an aqueous medium requires an expenditure of about 4 kcal of free energy. Hence the nonpolar contacts contribute to the stability of the structure and it is not too surprising that hemoglobin is sensitive to small alterations in the nonpolar contacts. Two types of contact between unlike chains are possible—$\alpha_1\beta_1$ (same as $\alpha_2\beta_2$) and $\alpha_1\beta_2$ (same as $\alpha_2\beta_1$). The two are distinguished on the basis of the specific residues that participate in the contact shown in

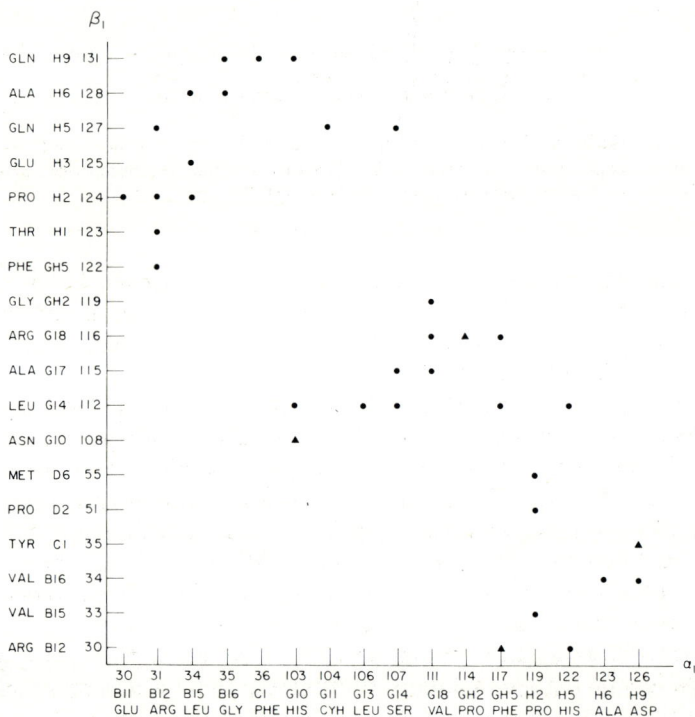

Fig. 2.7. The amino-acid residues that participate in the $\alpha_1\beta_1$ contact in horse oxyhemoglobin. Solid dots: van-der-Waals interactions; triangles: hydrogen bonds (PERUTZ, 1969a)

Figs. 2.7 and 2.8 and of the two, the $\alpha_1\beta_2$ contact is more deeply involved in the oxygenation process. Also, it is in the $\alpha_1\beta_2$ contact region (as well as in the contact region between the heme and the polypeptide chain) that we find the residues which are constant from one mammalian species to another.

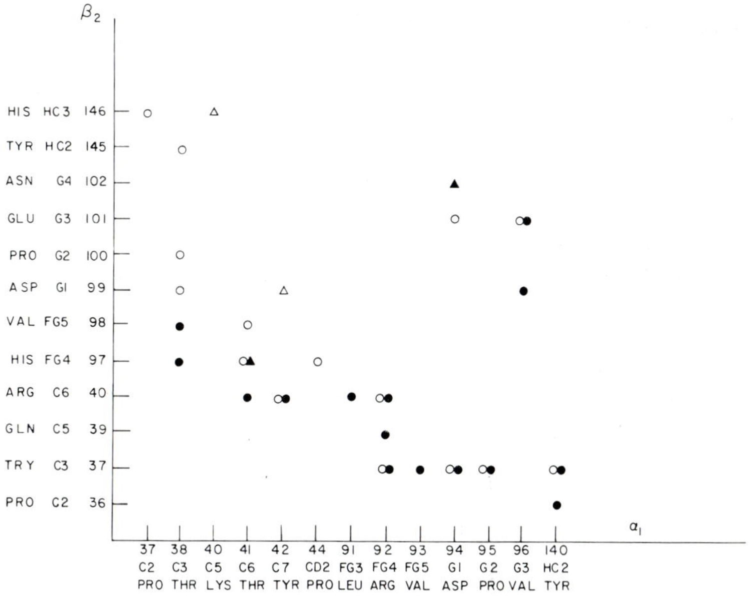

β_2

```
HIS HC3 146 ─   o         △
TYR HC2 145 ─       o
ASN  G4 102 ─                              ▲
GLU  G3 101 ─                         o        o●
PRO  G2 100 ─   o
ASP  G1  99 ─   o       △                        ●
VAL FG5  98 ─  ●     o
HIS FG4  97 ─  ●    o▲      o
ARG  C6  40 ─      ●  o●    ●  o●
GLN  C5  39 ─                  ●
TRY  C3  37 ─              o●  ●  o●  o●    o●
PRO  C2  36 ─                              ●
            └─┴──┴──┴──┴──┴──┴──┴──┴──┴──┴──┴──  α₁
              37 38 40 41 42 44 91 92 93 94 95 96 140
              C2 C3 C5 C6 C7 CD2 FG3 FG4 FG5 G1 G2 G3 HC2
              PRO THR LYS THR TYR PRO LEU ARG VAL ASP PRO VAL TYR
```

Fig. 2.8. The amino-acid residues that participate in the $\alpha_1\beta_2$ contact in horse hemoglobin. Open (solid) dots and triangles represent van-der-Waals interactions and hydrogen bonds respectively in deoxyhemoglobin (oxyhemoglobin) (PERUTZ, 1969a)

In addition to van-der-Waals interactions and hydrogen bonds there are also a number of salt bridges within and between subunits in deoxyhemoglobin. The ones that have an important bearing on the oxygenation characteristics of hemoglobin are the following (Fig. 2.9):

    1. α-carboxyl of arginine HC 3 (141 α_1)—α-amino of valine NA 2 (1 α_2);

    2. guanidinium of arginine HC 3 (141 α_1)—β-carboxyl of aspartate H 9 (126 α_2);

    3. ε-amino of lysine C 5 (40 α_1)—α-carboxyl of histidine HC 3 (146 β_2);

    4. imidazole of histidine HC 3 (146 β_1)—β-carboxyl of aspartate FG 1 (94 β_1).

Salt bridges are also obtained by interchanging α_1 with α_2 and β_1 with β_2. The salt bridges do not exist in oxyhemoglobin; the ends of each chain are therefore free and the structure is said to be "relaxed" (R), in contrast to deoxyhemoglobin, which is "constrained" or "tense" (T).

    The state of oxygenation has an important bearing on the relative positions and orientations of the four subunits. Fortunately, there is a fairly simple way of describing the relative motion of the subunits accompanying a change in oxygenation: If a coordinate system is placed with its origin at the center of mass of the four heme groups in oxyhemoglobin, the movement of the subunits upon

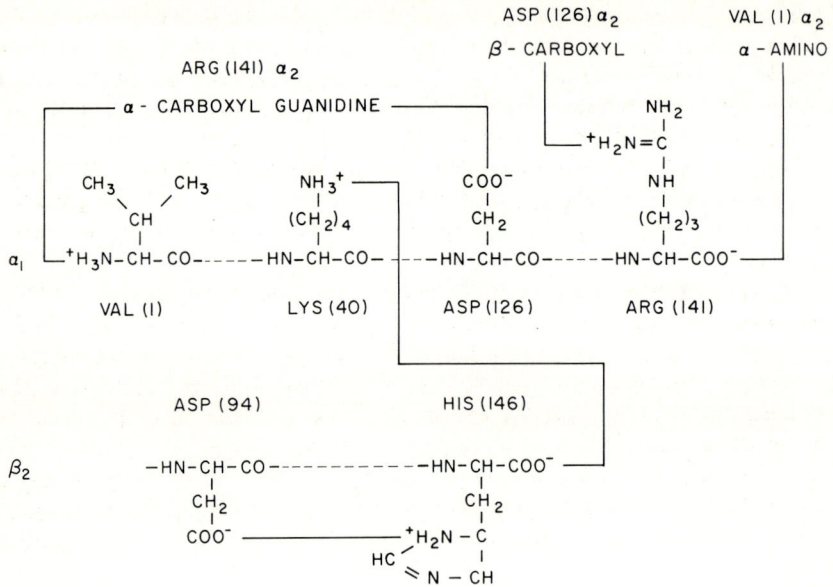

Fig. 2.9. Salt bridges in deoxyhemoglobin

deoxygenation can be described as simple rotations about certain axes fixed in the coordinate system. α chains rotate $9.4°$ and β chains $7.4°$, but they do not shift along the axes. The total motion of the center of mass is 1.4 Å for α chains and 2.9 Å for β chains.

These movements give rise to changes in the contact regions (Table 2.5). In T, the $\alpha_1\beta_1$ contacts involve 98 atoms from 32 residues as against 110 atoms from 34 residues in R. The $\alpha_1\beta_2$ contact involves 69 atoms from 20 residues in T and 110 atoms from 34 residues in R. The main difference, however, between $\alpha_1\beta_1$ and $\alpha_1\beta_2$ is that upon oxygenation the rotation between α_1 and β_1 is $4°$ and the shifts between atoms is less that 1 Å whereas the rotation between α_1 and β_2 is $13.5°$ and there are local displacements as large as 7 Å. Another impor-

Table 2.5. *Some properties of the contact regions between chains* (PERUTZ *et al.*, 1968 b)

Contact	Quaternary Conformation	Number of Residues	Number of Atoms	Effect of R−T transition	Remarks
$\alpha_1\alpha_2$	R, T				Very few contacts, some
$\beta_1\beta_2$	R, T				salt bridges and hydrogen bonds
$\alpha_1\beta_1$	R	34	110	Small changes in	Participating helices are
$\alpha_1\beta_1$	T	32	98	contact region	α(BGH)−β(HGB)
$\alpha_1\beta_2$	R	19	80	Large changes in	Participating helices are
$\alpha_1\beta_2$	T	20	69	contact region	α(CFG)−β(FCG)

tant characteristic of the $\alpha_1\beta_2$ contact is shown in Fig. 2.10 (MORIMOTO *et al.*, 1971): In the transition from T to R the hydrogen bond between tyrosine C 7 $(42\alpha_1)$ and aspartate G 1 $(99\beta_2)$ switches to a position between aspartate G 1 $(92\alpha_1)$ and asparagine G 4 $(102\beta_2)$. Hence there are two energetically stable positions and the contact can "click" into one or the other.

The movement of the subunits upon oxygenations also affects the distances between iron atoms (Table 2.4). The distance between Fe β_1 and Fe β_2 decreases from 39.9 to 33.4 Å while the Fe $\alpha_1 -$ Fe α_2 separation is slightly increased — from 34.9 to 36.0 Å.

We have already called attention to the fact that when a subunit becomes oxygenated and its tertiary structure switches from t to r, tyrosine HC 2 is expelled from its pocket and produces displacement of the C-terminal residue. The effect of this displacement is to rupture the salt bridges listed above, since all of them involve C-terminal residues; the latter then become free to rotate and the tyrosines attached to them acquire partial freedom.

The question often arises as to whether the structure of a molecule as revealed by X-ray diffraction on a single crystal is identical with the molecule in solution or in the physiological environment. It is, of course, impossible to give a totally

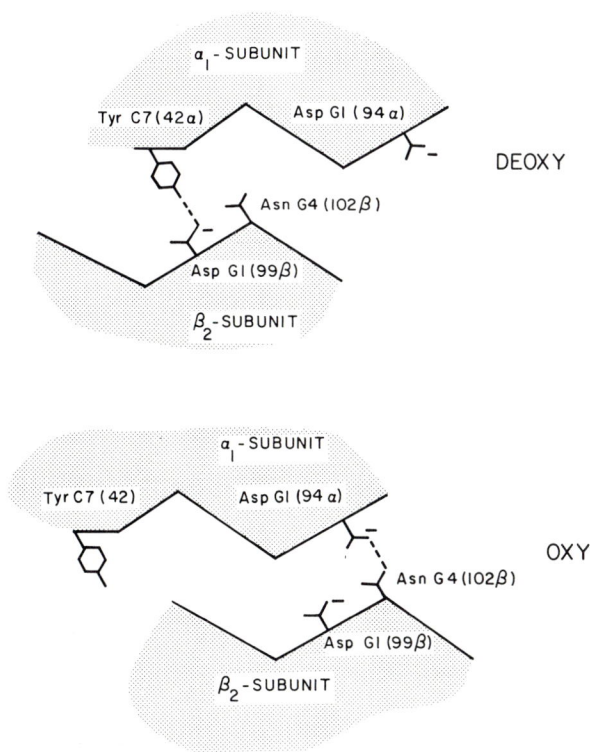

Fig. 2.10. The switching of a hydrogen bond in the $\alpha_1\beta_2$ contact on oxygenation. The contact "clicks" from one position to the other (MORIMOTO *et al.*, 1971)

unequivocal answer. However, all the available evidence, including magnetic resonance experiments which can be performed both on single crystals and in solution, point to the conclusion that there are no major differences in the conformations.

2.6 Dissociated Hemoglobin

Oxyhemoglobin dissociates into dimers over a wide range of conditions, such as low and high pH or in strong salt solution even at neutral pH. The $\alpha_1 \alpha_2 \beta_1 \beta_2$ tetramer splits into two $\alpha\beta$ dimers (not $\alpha_1 \alpha_2$ or $\beta_1 \beta_2$) and it is likely that the dimers are of the $\alpha_1 \beta_1$ type rather than the $\alpha_1 \beta_2$ type. Further dissociation of the dimers into free α and β chains is possible, though β chains have a tendency to form dimers ($\beta_1 \beta_2$) and tetramers ($\beta_1 \beta_2 \beta_3 \beta_4$) while α chains exist as monomers. The dissociation is reversible in that functional hemoglobin can be reformed from isolated α and β chains.

In sharp contrast, deoxyhemoglobin hardly dissociates. It has been estimated (KELLETT and GUTFREUND, 1970) that the rate of dissociation of deoxyhemoglobin is lower than that of oxyhemoglobin by a factor of at least 3×10^4.

Chapter III

Oxygenation Characteristics

3.1 Equilibrium Curves

The main physiological function of hemoglobin is to pick up molecular oxygen in the lungs, transport it to the tissues and deposit it there[2]. This it can do because the binding of oxygen to hemoglobin is reversible; that is, the overall reaction is described by the equation

$$Hb + 4 O_2 \rightleftharpoons Hb(O_2)_4 .$$

If the saturation, y, is defined as the ratio of the number of occupied to the total number of available oxygen binding sites, it is then possible to determine the dependence of y on the partial pressure of oxygen experimentally. Such a curve is shown in Fig. 3.1; it is known as an equilibrium or saturation curve. At the

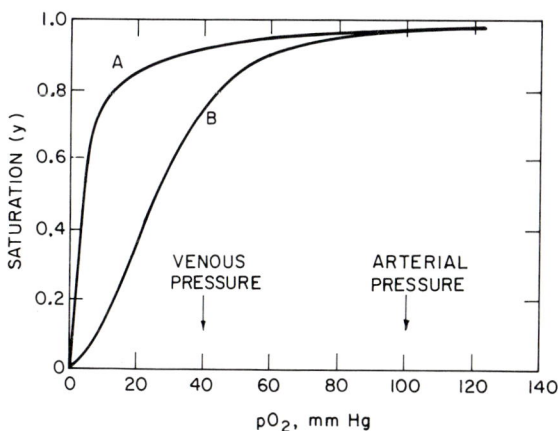

Fig. 3.1 A and B. Oxygen equilibrium curves of A myoglobin and B hemoglobin

partial pressures prevailing in the lungs (about 100 mm Hg), hemoglobin is almost totally saturated with oxygen, i.e. almost all the available binding sites are occupied by oxygen. At lower partial pressures, as in the tissues, much of the oxygen has been released and the saturation is consequently reduced.

---

[2] Hemoglobin also transports CO_2 but CO_2 is not bound to the heme group. The mechanism in therefore quite different from that of oxygen transport, although there are certain links between the two processes.

Myoglobin also binds oxygen reversibly but its dependence on oxygen pressure (Fig. 3.1) is quite different from that of hemoglobin. At pressures above about 80 mm Hg both myoglobin and hemoglobin are almost completely saturated. However, as the pressure is reduced, the saturation of hemoglobin falls much faster than that of myoglobin: At 20 mm Hg the saturation of hemoglobin is about 0.4 while in myoglobin it is about 0.85. This property of hemoglobin is a rather fortunate one for physiological purposes, because an oxygen carrier must not only bind oxygen but must also release it readily in order that the tissues be adequately supplied with oxygen. We see that hemoglobin has this property whereas myoglobin, though it binds oxygen quite easily, requires a much lower partial pressure before releasing it. Thus if myoglobin were the oxygen carrier, the tissues would suffer severely from lack of oxygen.

What is the origin of this difference? A large number and variety of experiments with dissociated hemoglobin provide convincing proof that the individual subunits which together make up the hemoglobin molecule do not of themselves behave differently from myoglobin. The difference between hemoglobin and myoglobin must, then, be associated with subunit interactions which somehow alter the shape of the equilibrium curve. This is a real, fundamental, difference in the behavior of the two molecules. The sigmoidal (S-shaped) curve in hemoglobin, in contrast to the hyperbolic curve of myoglobin, implies, as we shall see, the existence of a cooperative effect among the four subunits so that the detachment of oxygen from one subunit increases the probability of release of oxygen from another subunit of the same hemoglobin molecule. Similarly, the binding of oxygen to the heme group of one subunit has the effect of increasing the affinity of a neighboring subunit (on the same molecule) for oxygen. The extent of cooperativity among subunits can perhaps be appreciated through a remark of PERUTZ (1970), who pointed out that if we have two hemoglobin molecules A and B, with three sites on A bound to O_2 but all sites on B vacant then the probability of an approaching free oxygen molecule sticking to A is 70 times greater than the probability of its sticking to B. It is this cooperative behavior in hemoglobin in its reaction with oxygen which may be regarded as the central problem to which much of present-day research in hemoglobin is directed.

We have already noted that ferrohemoglobin may also bind other ligands, such as CO and NO. These are characterized by saturation curves whose shapes are very similar to the oxygen curve, although the positions of these curves along the pressure axis may be quite different. From the similarity in shape we conclude that subunit interactions which lead to cooperativity must be present, while the displacement along the pressure axis is an indication of the strength of binding or affinity of hemoglobin for that ligand. A numerical measure of affinity is $p_{1/2}$, the partial pressure of the gas when the saturation is 0.5. Another measure is the partition constant, a, defined for two gases such as CO and O_2 by

$$\frac{[HbCO]}{[HbO_2]} = a\frac{pCO}{pO_2}.$$

For these gases a lies in the range of 200 to 250, indication a far greater affinity of hemoglobin for carbon monoxide than for oxygen. Another point of interest is that the cooperative aspects of hemoglobin extend from one type of ligand to another. If, for instance, CO is bound to one subunit, the affinity of another subunit on the same molecule for O_2 (and CO) is increased. It appears that the crucial factor is whether the sixth position is occupied or vacant; the precise nature of the ligand is of lesser importance. Ferrihemoglobin, as mentioned earlier, also binds several ligands, but the binding is not cooperative.

There is an important parallel between the saturation properties of myoglobin and hemoglobin on the one hand and the velocity characteristics of certain enzymes on the other. For some enzyme-catalyzed reactions the velocity as a function of substrate concentration has the shape of a rectangular hyperbola similar to the saturation curve of myoglobin. In other enzymes the catalytic action is strongly influenced by interactions with small molecules whose binding sites are distinct and often distant from the binding sites for the substrate. The velocity characteristic of such an enzyme is frequently sigmoidal and, as in the case of hemoglobin, the origin of the sigmoidal characteristic is to be found in cooperative interactions within the molecule.

3.2 Quantitative Description

It is possible to give a more quantitative description of the saturation curves. This is particularly simple in the case of myoglobin, for which the equilibrium equation is

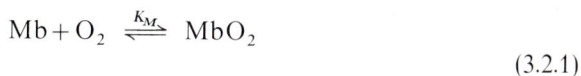

$$Mb + O_2 \overset{K_M}{\rightleftharpoons} MbO_2$$

with   (3.2.1)

$$K_M = \frac{[MbO_2]}{[Mb][O_2]}.$$

Since the concentration of occupied sites is the same as the concentration of MbO_2 while the concentration of all possible sites is equal to the sum of the concentrations of Mb and MbO_2, the fractional saturation is

$$y = \frac{[MbO_2]}{[Mb]+[MbO_2]} = \frac{K_M[O_2]}{1+K_M[O_2]}.$$

If we let x represent the concentration of oxygen, $[O_2]$, or equivalently the partial pressure, pO_2,

$$y = \frac{K_M x}{1+K_M x}.$$ (3.2.2)

This is the equation for a rectangular hyperbola and accurately describes the saturation of myoglobin. It is often useful to rewrite (3.2.2) as

$$H = \frac{y}{1-y} = K_M x,$$ (3.2.3)

and in this form it is known as the Hill equation.

As we have seen, the saturation curve for hemoglobin is more complicated; it has a sigmoidal shape and cannot be derived from any simple equilibrium relation analogous to (3.2.1). However, a good empirical relation for hemoglobin in the range 0.1—0.9 saturation is given by

$$y = \frac{K x^n}{1 + K x^n} \tag{3.2.4}$$

in which K and n are adjustable constants. The exponent n is known as the Hill constant; it is equal to 2.8—3.0, and is independent of pH and temperature. The Hill equation now takes the form

$$H = K x^n \tag{3.2.5}$$

or, in terms of experimental data it may be written

$$H = \left(\frac{p O_2}{p_{1/2}}\right)^n . \tag{3.2.5a}$$

An experimental curve of $\log H$ vs. $\log p O_2$ for hemoglobin, known as a Hill plot, is shown in Fig. 3.2; the Hill constant, n, is obtained directly from the slope in the midrange.

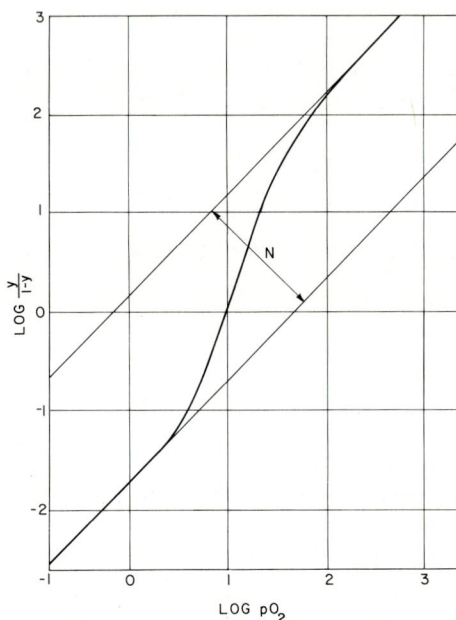

Fig. 3.2. Hill plot of the oxygen equilibrium of hemoglobin at pH 7. N is proportional to $\Delta G_1^l - \Delta G_4^l$ where ΔG_1^l and ΔG_4^l are the free energies of interaction associated with the binding of the first and last oxygen molecule, respectively

It is clear that these equations also describe the oxygenation of myoglobin, for it is only necessary to set $n = 1$ to obtain relations having the same form as (3.2.2) or (3.2.3).

To see the significance of n in greater detail we consider a macromolecule, M, with two binding sites for a ligand A. The equilibrium equations are

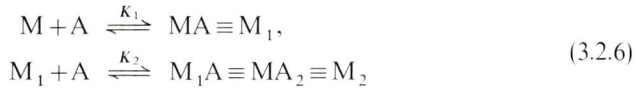

$$M+A \xrightleftharpoons{K_1} MA \equiv M_1,$$
$$M_1+A \xrightleftharpoons{K_2} M_1A \equiv MA_2 \equiv M_2 \tag{3.2.6}$$

with

$$K_1 = \frac{[M_1]}{[M][A]}, \quad K_2 = \frac{[M_2]}{[M_1][A]}. \tag{3.2.6a}$$

The saturation, in this case, is given by

$$2y = \frac{[M_1]+2[M_2]}{[M]+[M_1]+[M_2]} = \frac{K_1[A]+2K_1K_2[A]^2}{1+K_1[A]+K_1K_2[A]^2}. \tag{3.2.7}$$

If we let

$$a=[A], \quad C_1=K_1, \quad C_2=K_1K_2,$$

then

$$2y = \frac{C_1a+2C_2a^2}{1+C_1a+C_2a^2} = \frac{C_1a+2C_2a^2}{P(a)}. \tag{3.2.8}$$

Here, $P(a)$ is the polynomial in the denominator. The theory of partial fractions permits us to express the saturation function by

$$2y = \frac{a}{a-r_1} + \frac{a}{a-r_2} \tag{3.2.9}$$

in which r_1 and r_2 are the roots of $P(a)=0$. Setting

$$k_1 = -1/r_1, \quad k_2 = -1/r_2$$

we get

$$2y = \frac{k_1a}{1+k_1a} + \frac{k_2a}{1+k_2a}. \tag{3.2.10}$$

It is instructive to obtain (3.2.10) by another method which is rather better suited to the interpretation of k_1 and k_2. Let us suppose that the two binding sites on M are not equivalent and that different equilibrium constants govern the binding of A to the two sites. This means that when there is only a single ligand attached to M, there are two cases, which might be represented by M'A and M"A. The equilibrium equations for the reaction of M with A take the form (EDSALL and WYMAN, 1958)

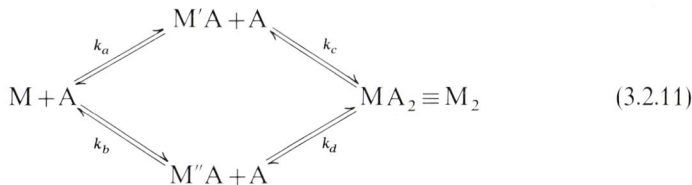

$$\tag{3.2.11}$$

where

$$k_a = \frac{[\text{M}'\text{A}]}{[\text{M}][\text{A}]}, \qquad k_b = \frac{[\text{M}''\text{A}]}{[\text{M}][\text{A}]},$$

$$k_c = \frac{[\text{M}_2]}{[\text{M}'\text{A}][\text{A}]}, \qquad k_d = \frac{[\text{M}_2]}{[\text{M}''\text{A}][\text{A}]}. \qquad (3.2.12)$$

The constants k_a, k_b, k_c and k_d are known as the microscopic or intrinsic equilibrium constants. They are not all independent since, from (3.2.12)

$$k_a k_c = k_b k_d. \qquad (3.2.13)$$

Since M_1 in (3.2.6) is a single-ligand molecule, with no distinction as to which of the two possible sites is occupied, we have, for the concentrations

$$[\text{M}_1] \equiv [\text{MA}] = [\text{M}'\text{A}] + [\text{M}''\text{A}]. \qquad (3.2.14)$$

The connections between K_1 and K_2 defined in (3.2.6a) and the microscopic constants are readily obtained from (3.2.12) and (3.2.14). They are

$$K_1 = k_a + k_b,$$

$$\frac{1}{K_2} = \frac{1}{k_c} + \frac{1}{k_d}. \qquad (3.2.15)$$

The saturation function (3.2.7) can now also be expressed in terms of the microscopic constants, and upon setting $k_a = k_c = k_1$ and $k_b = k_d = k_2$ we obtain (3.2.10). However we cannot stop here because (3.2.13) must also be taken into account so that k_1 and k_2 are not independent, but $k_1 = \pm k_2$. The negative sign leads to a negative saturation which has no physical meaning. Hence, if $k_1 = k_2 = k$, (3.2.10) becomes

$$y = \frac{k_a}{1 + k_a}. \qquad (3.2.16)$$

In the interpretation of (3.2.16), we note that the equilibrium equations (3.2.11) imply that if the two binding sites on M are indistinguishable, then $k_a = k_b$. From (3.2.13) we must also have $k_c = k_d$. If in addition, there is no interaction between the sites, k_a, k_b, k_c and k_d are all equal to a common value k and the saturation is given by (3.2.16). The latter is of the same form as (3.2.2); hence the Hill equation must have the same form as (3.2.3), i.e.

$$H = ka \qquad (3.2.17)$$

with the Hill constant $n = 1$. Finally, for this case we have, from (3.2.15)

$$K_1 = 2k,$$

$$K_2 = \frac{k}{2}. \qquad (3.2.18)$$

It is seen that two equivalent (indistinguishable) binding sites which are independent (non-interacting) are characterized by equations (3.2.16, 17 and 18). [It will shortly be shown that (3.2.16) and (3.2.17) are valid for any number of equivalent, independent binding sites].

Let us now suppose that the two binding sites cooperate strongly though they are still assumed to be equivalent. The latter condition, as we have seen above, implies that $k_a = k_b$ and $k_c = k_d$. Also from (3.2.15)

$$K_1 = 2k_a,$$
$$K_2 = \frac{k_c}{2} \qquad\qquad (3.2.19)$$

and the saturation function (3.2.7) is

$$y = \frac{k_a a(1 + k_c a)}{1 + k_a a(2 + k_c a)}. \qquad\qquad (3.2.20)$$

The assumption of strong cooperativity means that whenever a single ligand is bound to M to form M_1, the probability of binding the second ligand is greatly increased, resulting in the formation of M_2. Therefore, under equilibrium, the concentration of M_1 will be much smaller than that of M_2. From (3.2.12) for $[M_2] \gg [M_1]$, where M_1 is given by (3.2.14),

$$k_c a \gg 1. \qquad\qquad (3.2.21)$$

Therefore

$$y = \frac{k_a k_c a^2}{1 + k_a k_c a^2} = \frac{C_2 a^2}{1 + C_2 a^2} \qquad\qquad (3.2.22)$$

and

$$H = C_2 a^2. \qquad\qquad (3.2.23)$$

The Hill constant in this case is 2 and this is its maximum value for a macromolecule with two binding sites. We conclude, therefore, that a positive (cooperative) interaction between two binding sites manifests itself through the relation

$$1 < n < 2.$$

A simple extension of (3.2.8) to q sites gives

$$qy = \frac{C_1 a + 2C_2 a^2 + \cdots + qC_q a^q}{P(a)} = \frac{k_1 a}{1 + k_1 a} + \cdots + \frac{k_q a}{1 + k_q a} \qquad (3.2.24)$$

where

$$P(a) = 1 + C_1 a + \cdots + C_q a^q,$$
$$C_i = K_1 K_2 \ldots K_i,$$
$$k_i = -\frac{1}{r_i}. \qquad\qquad (3.2.24\,a)$$

The quantities r_i are the roots of $P(a) = 0$. FLETCHER et al. (1970) discuss the general case including the occurrence of complex roots; for our purpose it is assumed that the r_i are real. From the definition of the C_i, it is seen that they may be interpreted as equilibrium constants associated with the reaction

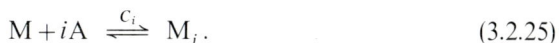

$$M + iA \xrightleftharpoons{C_i} M_i. \qquad\qquad (3.2.25)$$

Eq. (3.2.24) can also be written $(C_0=1)$

$$qy = \frac{\displaystyle\sum_{i=0}^{q} i C_i a^i}{\displaystyle\sum_{i=0}^{q} C_i a^i} = \frac{d\ln \displaystyle\sum_{i=0}^{q} C_i a^i}{d\ln a}. \tag{3.2.26}$$

This is the form employed by WYMAN (1964), who also introduced the terminology of binding polynomial or binding potential for $RT \ln P(a)$. If the binding sites are all alike and independent of one another it is possible, as before, to express the saturation function in terms of a single microscopic constant. For such a case

$$P(a)=(1+ka)^q$$

and
$$\tag{3.2.27}$$

$$y = \frac{ka}{1+ka}.$$

It must nevertheless be pointed out, as WYMAN did (1968), that a combination of positive (cooperative) interactions and unlike sites could, in principle, produce relationships of the same form as (3.2.27). However, in the absence of other evidence the assumption of independent, identical sites would be the most natural one. When there are four binding sites, as in hemoglobin

$$\begin{aligned}
K_1 &= 4k, & C_1 &= 4k, \\
K_2 &= \tfrac{3}{2}k, & C_2 &= 6k^2, \\
K_3 &= \tfrac{2}{3}k, & C_3 &= 4k^3, \\
K_4 &= \tfrac{1}{4}k, & C_4 &= k^4.
\end{aligned} \tag{3.2.28}$$

As in the previous case, the assumption of maximum cooperativity leads to a value of n equal to the number of binding sites; for hemoglobin this would be 4.

3.3 The Bohr Effect

The affinity of hemoglobin for oxygen depends on pH; this is the oxygen Bohr effect. Fig. 3.3 shows two equilibrium curves for human hemoglobin, one at pH 7 and the other at pH 9.1; the curves are very similar in shape but are displaced from each other along the pressure axis and therefore have different values for $p_{1/2}$. They illustrate the difference in affinity at the two pH values, but since the shapes of the equilibrium curves are not altered, the cooperative characteristics are not affected by a change in pH[3]. Over a wider range of pH the affinity of hemoglobin for oxygen, as measured by $p_{1/2}$, varies as shown in Fig. 3.4. The curve has a maximum at about pH 6.5, which is the pH corresponding to minimum oxygen affinity. Since physiological pH is 7.4, the region of interest lies in the alkaline (high pH) side of the maximum and in this region a reduction of pH (increase in proton concentration) increases $p_{1/2}$. This signifies that the

---

[3] It has recently been observed that there is a small decrease in the Hill constant (n) as the pH is increased (TYUMA, I., KAMIGAWARA, Y., IMAI, K.: pH Dependence of the Shape of the Hemoglobin-Oxygen Equilibrium Curve. Biochim. Biophys. Acta **310**, 317—320 (1973)).

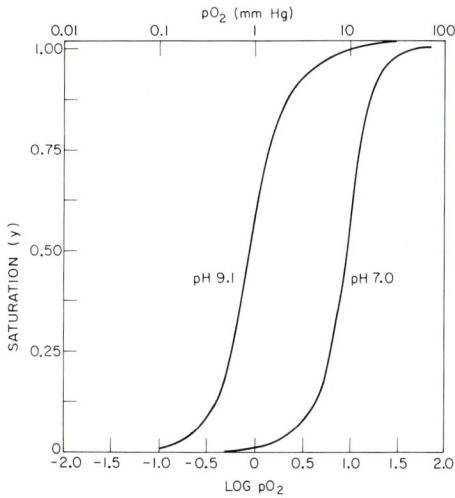

Fig. 3.3. The effect of pH on oxygen equilibrium curves

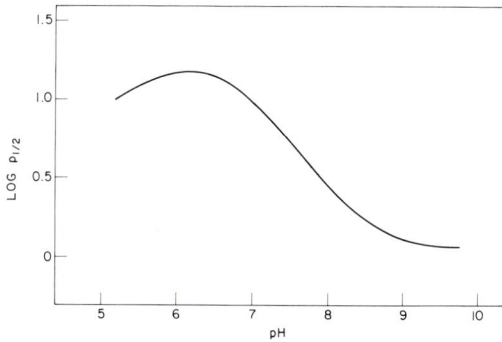

Fig. 3.4. Effect of pH on the affinity of hemoglobin for oxygen

saturation curve has been displaced to higher pressures and that the affinity has been reduced. Alternatively, it may be said that a reduction in affinity is equivalent to a shift in the equilibrium concentrations of oxy- and deoxyhemoglobin in the direction of the latter.

Another way to view the Bohr effect is to recognize that oxyhemoglobin is a stronger acid (proton donor) than deoxyhemoglobin. The alkaline Bohr effect therefore associates the binding of oxygen with the release of protons or conversely, the removal of protons will increase the affinity for oxygen, since the relationship must be a reciprocal one. Furthermore, there is a proportionality between the number of protons released and the number of oxygen molecules that are bound. At physiological pH, for example, the proportionality constant is about 0.6 protons per oxygen molecule. On the face of it, the existence of a relationship between the release of protons and the binding of oxygen is rather strange, since the only source of protons are certain amino acids which contain ionizable side chains, and these are distinct from the heme groups which are the binding sites for oxygen.

The binding of other ligands like CO or NO to ferrohemoglobin is also accompanied by a Bohr effect. However there is no Bohr effect associated with the binding of ligands to ferrihemoglobin, nor does it exist in myoglobin or in isolated α or β chains. These experimental observations provide a strong suggestion that cooperativity and the Bohr effect must be related to one another in some way.

The Bohr effect can be discussed in a more quantitative fashion by means of the formalism of linked functions introduced by WYMAN (1964). Let us suppose that a macromolecule is capable of binding q ligands of a type A and p ligands of type B. By analogy with (3.2.25), the equilibrium equations are

$$M + iA + jB \underset{}{\overset{C_{ij}}{\rightleftharpoons}} M_{ij}. \qquad (3.3.1)$$

The fractional saturation by ligand A is defined, as usual, as the ratio of the number of sites occupied by A to the total number of binding sites available to A. It is therefore given by

$$q y_A = \frac{\sum\limits_{i=0}^{q} \sum\limits_{j=0}^{p} i[M_{ij}]}{\sum\limits_{i=0}^{q} \sum\limits_{j=0}^{p} [M_{ij}]}. \qquad (3.3.2)$$

From (3.3.1)

$$C_{ij} = \frac{[M_{ij}]}{[M] a^i b^j} \qquad (3.3.3)$$

where $a = [A]$ and $b = [B]$. Combination of (3.3.2) and (3.3.3) gives

$$q y_A = \frac{\sum\limits_{i=0}^{q} \sum\limits_{j=0}^{p} i C_{ij} a^i b^j}{\sum\limits_{i=0}^{q} \sum\limits_{j=0}^{p} C_{ij} a^i b^j}. \qquad (3.3.4)$$

A more compact form of (3.3.4) is obtained by defining a function

$$S = \sum\limits_{i=0}^{q} \sum\limits_{j=0}^{p} C_{ij} a^i b^j. \qquad (3.3.5)$$

It may then be verified by direct differentiation that

$$q y_A = \frac{\partial \ln S}{\partial \ln a}. \qquad (3.3.6)$$

Similarly,

$$p y_B = \frac{\partial \ln S}{\partial \ln b}. \qquad (3.3.7)$$

Differentiating (3.3.6) and (3.3.7)

$$q \left(\frac{\partial y_A}{\partial \ln b} \right)_a = p \left(\frac{\partial y_B}{\partial \ln a} \right)_b. \qquad (3.3.8)$$

This is WYMAN's fundamental linkage equation. Other relations among the variable are readily obtained; thus from

$$dy_A = \left(\frac{\partial y_A}{\partial \ln a}\right)_b d\ln a + \left(\frac{\partial y_A}{\partial \ln b}\right)_a d\ln b$$

we obtain, for y_A kept constant,

$$q\left(\frac{\partial \ln a}{\partial \ln b}\right)_{y_A} = -p\left(\frac{\partial y_B}{\partial y_A}\right)_b. \tag{3.3.9}$$

Similarly, when y_B is kept constant,

$$q\left(\frac{\partial \ln a}{\partial \ln b}\right)_{y_B} = -p\left(\frac{\partial y_B}{\partial y_A}\right)_a. \tag{3.3.10}$$

If, now, we make the identifications

$$y_A = y = \text{oxygen saturation},$$
$$y_B = [H^+] = \text{proton saturation},$$
$$a = pO_2 = \text{partial pressure of oxygen},$$
$$-\log b = \text{pH}$$

then (3.3.8) becomes

$$q\left(\frac{\partial y}{\partial \text{pH}}\right)_{pO_2} = p\left(\frac{\partial [H^+]}{\partial \log p O_2}\right)_{\text{pH}}. \tag{3.3.11}$$

This implies that if an increase in oxygen activity (or concentration, or partial pressure) at constant pH has the effect of increasing the dissociation of protons ($[H^+]$ reduced), then the right-hand side of (3.3.11) is positive and an increase in pH should produce an increase in oxygen saturation at constant oxygen activity. Another useful relation is obtained from (3.3.9), and can be written

$$\left(\frac{\partial \log p_{1/2}}{\partial \text{pH}}\right)_{y=0.5} = \Delta[H^+] \tag{3.3.12}$$

where $\Delta[H^+] = [H^+]$ (oxyhemoglobin) $- [H^+]$ (deoxyhemoglobin) is the difference in the number of protons bound by oxy- and deoxyhemoglobin per oxygen binding site.

In addition to a dependence on pH, the binding of oxygen to hemoglobin is influenced by other factors. Thus, an increase in temperature will shift the equilibrium curve along the pressure axis in the direction of higher pressures; an increase of 10 °C, for example, will decrease the affinity by a factor of approximately 2, but the shape of the curve remains essentially unaltered. This implies that the cooperative effect is independent of temperature and suggests that the mechanism, whatever it is, involves entropic rather than energetic changes.

When hemoglobin is dissociated into dimers by extremes in pH or salt concentration, the oxygen-binding characteristics are essentially unchanged; indeed the Hill constant remains at the tetrameric value of approximately 3. This at first seemed paradoxical since n cannot exceed the number of binding sites.

However, as has been noted previously (Section 2.6), it is only oxyhemoglobin that dissociates, whereas deoxyhemoglobin remains practically intact. Hence the equilibrium curve that is observed is still that of the tetramer and it is only after the tetramer has become oxygenated that dissociation takes place. Isolated α and β chains, β dimers, and tetramers all have the capacity to bind oxygen; in fact, the affinity is as high or higher than in the tetramer but the equilibrium curve is hyperbolic ($n=1$) and there is no Bohr effect. More recently it has been shown (HEWITT et al., 1972) that $\alpha_1 \beta_1$ dimers which are products of the dissociation of oxyhemoglobin (Section 2.6) also have a high affinity for oxygen but are totally lacking in cooperative effects. It would appear, then, that the tetrameric molecule is the essential functional unit with cooperative characteristics.

Still another influence on the oxygenation process is that of DPG (2,3 diphosphoglycerate)[4], which binds strongly to deoxyhemoglobin but hardly at all to oxyhemoglobin. DPG is normally present in red cells and has the effect of causing the release of oxygen to occur at higher pressures, or it reduces the oxygen affinity, which amounts to the same thing, without, however, affecting the cooperative properties. We may see, now, the sense of a remark by PERUTZ (1970), that hemoglobin may be regarded as an enzyme with oxygen as the substrate, heme as the coenzyme and H^+ and DPG as allosteric effectors.

3.4 Thermodynamic and Kinetic Properties

The Hill plot (Fig. 3.2), whose slope in the midrange provides a measure for cooperativity, also contains information on the free energy of interaction among subunits when hemoglobin becomes fully oxygenated. This was shown by WYMAN (1964, 1967); a more recent derivation leading to somewhat different conclusions has been given by SAROFF and MINTON (1972), whose version we now summarize.

When the binding sites do not interact we have, from (3.2.28)

$$K_i = \frac{k}{\gamma_i},$$

$$\gamma_1 = \tfrac{1}{4}, \qquad \gamma_2 = \tfrac{2}{3}, \qquad \gamma_3 = \tfrac{3}{2}, \qquad \gamma_4 = 4 .$$

The free energy of binding of a molecule of oxygen is

$$\Delta G_0 = -R T \ln k = -R T \gamma_i K_i \tag{3.4.1}$$

_____

[4] 2,3 diphosphoglycerate

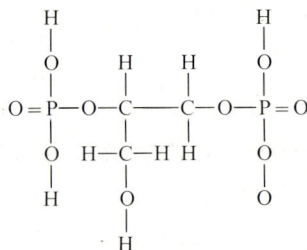

and is the same for any oxygen whether it is the first or last to be bound. On the other hand, when subunit interactions are present, the free energy of binding of an oxygen molecule depends on how many oxygens have previously been bound to the hemoglobin molecule. If we let ΔG_i be the free energy of binding of each successive oxygen, then in place of (3.4.1) we write

$$\Delta G_i = -R T \ln k + \Delta G_i^I \tag{3.4.2}$$

in which ΔG_i^I represents the free energy of interaction associated with the binding of the i-th oxygen. It is convenient to express (3.4.2) in the form

$$\Delta G_i = -R T \ln \gamma_i K_i^I \tag{3.4.3}$$

where

$$K_i^I = \frac{k}{\gamma} e^{-\Delta G_i^I / RT}$$

so that (3.4.3) formally resembles (3.4.1). Replacing K_i in (3.2.14 a) by K_i^I defines C_i^I; these quantities then replace the C_i in (3.2.14), from which a new Hill function is obtained. With $q=4$, $a=x=[O_2]$, the result is

$$H = \frac{S_1 k x + 3 S_2 k^2 x^2 + 3 S_3 k^3 x^3 + S_4 k^4 x^4}{1 + 3 S_1 k x + 3 S_2 k^2 x^2 + S_3 k^3 x^3} \tag{3.4.4}$$

where

$$S_i = \exp\left[-\sum_{r=1}^{i} \Delta G_r^I / R T \right].$$

We note that at low oxygen pressure (x small)

$$\log H = \log S_1 k x = \log H_S \tag{3.4.5}$$

while at high oxygen pressure (x large)

$$\log H = \log \frac{S_4}{S_3} k x = \log H_L. \tag{3.4.6}$$

It is seen that both $\log H_S$ and $\log H_L$ are linear in $\log x$ (or $\log p O_2$) and have unit slope. This is illustrated in Fig. 3.2 where $\log H$ is plotted against $\log p O_2$. However, the two lines are displaced from each other, and in the midrange the slope, which is the Hill constant, is approximately 3. If N is the perpendicular distance between the two lines,

$$N = \frac{1}{\sqrt{2}} [\log H_L - \log H_S] = \frac{1}{\sqrt{2}} \left[\log \frac{S_4}{S_1 S_3} \right] = \frac{1}{2.303 \sqrt{2} R T} [\Delta G_1^I - \Delta G_4^I]$$

or

$$\Delta G_1^I - \Delta G_4^I = 2.303 \sqrt{2} R T N. \tag{3.4.7}$$

In WYMAN's original treatment $2.303\sqrt{2} R T N$ was identified with the average free energy of interaction defined as

$$\overline{\Delta G_1} = \tfrac{1}{4} \sum_i \Delta G_i^I. \tag{3.4.8}$$

But, as pointed out by SAROFF and MINTON, the Hill plot yields (3.4.7), which is insufficient for the calculation of ΔG_I unless one assumes a model for the subunit interactions. We may nevertheless obtain an estimate of $\overline{\Delta G_I}$ by comparing the free energy change of hemoglobin upon oxygenation with the free energy change of isolated subunits upon oxygenation. These values may be obtained, for example, from the discussion of thermodynamic parameters by GUIDOTTI (1971) where we find -24 kcal/mole for the oxygenation of hemoglobin and -32 kcal/mole for the oxygenation of subunits, i.e.

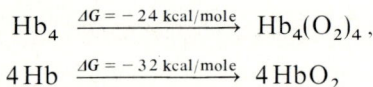

$$\mathrm{Hb_4} \xrightarrow{\Delta G = -24\ \mathrm{kcal/mole}} \mathrm{Hb_4(O_2)_4}\,,$$

$$4\,\mathrm{Hb} \xrightarrow{\Delta G = -32\ \mathrm{kcal/mole}} 4\,\mathrm{HbO_2}$$

where $\mathrm{Hb_4}$ is the tetramer and Hb is a single subunit. The average free energy of interaction, $\overline{\Delta G_I}$, may therefore be estimated as 8 kcal/mole of hemoglobin.

The general picture that emerges from this is that free energy is liberated when oxygen is bound to heme but part of it is expended in subunit interactions. PERUTZ (1970) points out that ΔG_I is comparable to the sum of the bond energies (6—12 kcal/mole) of the six interchain salt bridges—4 between α_1 and α_2 and one each in the $\alpha_1 \beta_2$ and $\alpha_2 \beta_1$ contacts (Section 2.5). Taken together with other stereochemical evidence, this makes it plausible to suppose that when hemoglobin becomes oxygenated, $\overline{\Delta G_I}$ is mainly expended in rupturing the salt bridges. On this basis, the salt bridges must make a significant contribution to the cooperative aspects of oxygenation (see, however, Section 4.5).

The kinetics of hemoglobin oxygenation and deoxygenation are far from simple, and a great deal remains to be explained. We shall confine our remarks to a few numerical values which appear to be reasonably well-established; a more detailed account is given by ANTONINI and BRUNORI (1970, 1971).

It is generally convenient for the purpose of kinetics to invoke the Adair scheme, which is based on the set of four sequential equilibria

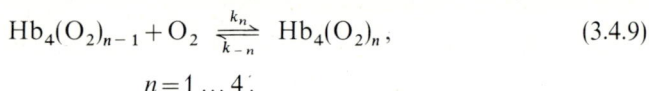

$$\mathrm{Hb_4(O_2)}_{n-1} + \mathrm{O_2} \underset{k_{-n}}{\overset{k_n}{\rightleftharpoons}} \mathrm{Hb_4(O_2)}_n\,, \tag{3.4.9}$$

$$n = 1 \ldots 4\,.$$

The constants k_n and k_{-n}—also known as "on" and "off" or combination and dissociation constants respectively—derive their meaning from the rate equations,

$$\frac{d}{dt}[\mathrm{Hb_4(O_2)}] = k_n[\mathrm{Hb_4(O_2)}_{n-1}][\mathrm{O_2}] - k_{-n}[\mathrm{Hb_4(O_2)}_n]\,. \tag{3.4.10}$$

The values of k_n and k_{-n} according to GIBSON (1970) are listed in Table 3.1 but it is well to bear in mind GIBSON's comment that "the basic scheme represented by the Adair equations is, in all likelihood, an over-simplification and the constants, though they give a good fit to the equilibrium curves are not necessarily unique". More recently, GIBSON (1973) has found large differences between α and β subunits in their reaction with oxygen—a result which casts even more doubt on the validity of (3.4.9).

It is often useful to have apparent kinetic constants which represent the overall reaction of hemoglobin with oxygen under certain specified conditions.

Thus, at 50% saturation $(y=0.5)$, the rate of combination is expressible by

$$\frac{d}{dt}[HbO_2]=k_{on}[Hb][O_2] \tag{3.4.11}$$

with $k_{on}=4.7 \times 10^6 \, M^{-1} \, sec^{-1}$ at 20 °C and pH 7 (ANTONINI and BRUNORI, 1971).

Table 3.1. *Kinetic constants for the oxygenation of hemoglobin based on the Adair scheme* (GIBSON, 1970)

	Phosphate buffer	Phosphate-free medium
	$M^{-1} \, sec^{-1}$	$M^{-1} \, sec^{-1}$
k_1	1.77×10^7	1.47×10^7
k_2	3.32	3.52
k_3	0.49	1.58
k_4	3.3	3.3
	sec^{-1}	sec^{-1}
k_{-1}	1900	136
k_{-2}	158	15.7
k_{-3}	539	138
k_{-4}	50	50

The dissociation of oxyhemoglobin, after the reaction is about 40% complete, can be represented by

$$\frac{d}{dt}[HbO_2]=-k_{off}[HbO_2] \tag{3.4.12}$$

with $k_{off}=35 \, sec^{-1}$ at 20 °C and pH 7 (DALZIEL and O'BRIEN, 1961). In addition, k_{off} (a) decreases as the pH is increased, (b) increases as the concentration of DPG is increased and (c) has a temperature dependence which can be described by an activation energy of 22 kcal/mole at pH 6.3 and 26 kcal/mole at pH 8.4.

Chapter IV

Approaches to Cooperativity

The central problem in the study of hemoglobin is to understand the mechanism of cooperativity, which manifests itself primarily in the sigmoidal saturation characteristic and the Bohr effect. At the outset we recognize that the matter cannot be simple because the iron atoms are separated by distances of 25 to 40 Å, which are much too great for direct (e.g. electromagnetic) interactions to be effective. In this chapter we discuss two general approaches toward the goal of understanding cooperativity in hemoglobin. The first one is thermodynamic in content and is based on a set of equilibrium equations constructed under a particular set of assumptions. In this category are the models proposed by MONOD et al., (1965) and by KOSHLAND et al., (1966). A rather different approach—one which seeks to understand cooperativity on the basis of the conformational differences between oxy- and deoxyhemoglobin—was employed by PERUTZ (1970, 1972).

4.1 The Monod-Wyman-Changeux (MWC) Model

The model proposed by MONOD et al. (1965) was devised primarily for allosteric proteins, in an attempt to explain the cooperativity observed in the behavior of certain enzymes. Though the model lends itself to a number of variations, we shall describe only the simplest version so that the main ideas do not become obscured by excessive detail. The basic assumptions are:

1. No distinction is made between α and β subunits.
2. There are two quaternary conformations, R and T.
3. Both forms can bind up to four molecules of O_2.
4. Subunits in R and T have different affinities for oxygen.
5. In each conformation there is a series of stepwise equilibria:

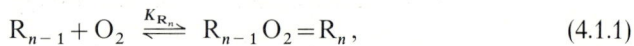

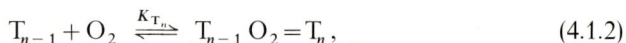

$$R_{n-1} + O_2 \xrightleftharpoons{K_{R_n}} R_{n-1}O_2 = R_n, \tag{4.1.1}$$

$$T_{n-1} + O_2 \xrightleftharpoons{K_{T_n}} T_{n-1}O_2 = T_n, \tag{4.1.2}$$

$$n = 1 \dots 4.$$

6. The constants $K_{R_1} \dots K_{R_4}$ can all be expressed in terms of a single microscopic constant k_R; similarly $K_{T_1} \dots K_{T_4}$ are expressible in terms of another microscopic constant, k_T. This implies that in each conformation the binding of oxygen is noncooperative, i.e. the probability of binding oxygen at a particular subunit

is independent of the state of oxygenation in the other subunits of the same molecule.

7. There is an equilibrium between the R and T forms:

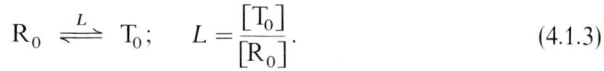

$$R_0 \xrightleftharpoons{L} T_0; \qquad L = \frac{[T_0]}{[R_0]}. \tag{4.1.3}$$

Under these assumptions we can derive a saturation function. From (3.2.24) and (3.2.28)

$$4y = \frac{[R_0](C_{R_1}x + \cdots + 4C_{R_4}x^4) + [T_0](C_{T_1}x + \cdots + 4C_{T_4}x^4)}{[R_0](1 + C_{R_1}x + \cdots + C_{R_4}x^4) + [T_0](1 + C_{T_1}x + \cdots + C_{T_4}x^4)} \tag{4.1.4}$$

where

$$\begin{aligned}
x &= [O_2], \\
C_{R_1} &= K_{R_1} = 4k_R, \\
C_{R_2} &= K_{R_1}K_{R_2} = 6k_R^2, \\
C_{R_3} &= K_{R_1}K_{R_2}K_{R_3} = 4k_R^3, \\
C_{R_4} &= K_{R_1}K_{R_2}K_{R_3}K_{R_4} = k_R^4.
\end{aligned} \tag{4.1.5}$$

Replacement of the index R by T in (4.1.5) gives the analogous expressions for $C_{T_1} \ldots C_{T_4}$. With

$$c = \frac{k_T}{k_R}, \qquad \alpha = k_R x, \tag{4.1.6}$$

we have, upon substituting (4.1.5) into (4.1.4)

$$y = \frac{Lc\alpha(1 + c\alpha)^3 + \alpha(1 + \alpha)^3}{L(1 + c\alpha)^4 + \alpha(1 + \alpha)^4}. \tag{4.1.7}$$

MONOD et al. (1965) obtained a good fit to hemoglobin equilibrium curves with $L = 9000$ and $c = 0.014$. But it should be noted that this is not a unique set of values; indeed the range of L appears to be $10^3 - 3 \times 10^5$ with a corresponding range for c of 0.04—0.001.

We can get a feeling for the manner in which cooperativity is built into the model. A high value of L implies that deoxygenated hemoglobin exists mainly in the T form, but a small value of c means that $k_T \ll k_R$ or that oxygen binds more readily to the R form. Thus, as R subunits become oxygenated, many more subunits must transform from T to R in order to maintain L constant, which means that more R molecules become available for oxygenation.

4.2 The Koshland-Nemethy-Filmer (KNF) Model

Like the previous one, the KNF model (KOSHLAND et al., 1966) treats α and β subunits as if they were alike. However, unlike the MWC model, it assumes that when a particular subunit becomes oxygenated, there is a change in the probability of oxygenation of a neighboring subunit. Presumably the interaction involves conformational changes, though this assumption is not an intrinsic part of the model. However, when so interpreted, the model postulates that the conformation of a subunit depends only on the presence or absence of an axial ligand on that subunit. This, then, agrees with the X-ray description (section 2.4).

The mathematics of the KNF model may be expressed in terms of equilibrium equations, by an analogous procedure to that followed in the last section. An alternative development was given by THOMPSON (1968) who employed the language of the Ising model in the theory of magnetism (see, for example, ZIMAN, 1965). The formalism of the Ising model is quite flexible and has been found to have applications beyond those in solid-state physics. We shall describe THOMPSON's development of the KNF model. The following definitions are employed:

$$\mu_i = \begin{cases} +1, & \text{subunit } i \text{ oxygenated}, \\ -1, & \text{subunit } i \text{ deoxygenated}. \end{cases}$$

Since there are four subunits, $i=1,2,3,4$. A configuration $\{\mu\}$ is defined by

$$\{\mu\} = \{\mu_1, \mu_2, \mu_3, \mu_4\}.$$

Thus, $\{\mu\}=\{1, 1, -1, 1\}$ describes a tetramer in which subunits 1, 2 and 4 are oxygenated and 3 is deoxygenated. In hemoglobin there can be 16 configurations corresponding to the two possible forms of each of the four subunits. $p(\mu_i)$ is the probability that subunit i is in the state of oxygenation described by the variable μ_i. For any subunit

$$p(+1)+p(-1)=1 \tag{4.2.1}$$

since every subunit must be in either the oxy- or the deoxy- state. It is mathematically convenient to define

$$p(\mu_i) = \frac{e^{\mu_i J}}{e^J + e^{-J}} = \frac{e^{\mu_i J}}{2\cosh J}. \tag{4.2.2}$$

In this form, $p(\mu_i)$ automatically satisfies (4.2.1). We define

$$\alpha = \frac{p(+1)}{p(-1)} = e^{2J}. \tag{4.2.3}$$

$P\{\mu\}$ is the probability of a configuration. Since the tetramer must reside in one of the possible configurations,

$$\sum_{\{\mu\}} P\{\mu\} = 1. \tag{4.2.4}$$

$N\{\mu\}$ is the number of subunits in a configuration that are oxygenated. It may be verified that

$$N\{\mu\} = 2 + \frac{1}{2}\sum_{i=1}^{4} \mu_i. \tag{4.2.5}$$

For example, when $\{\mu\} = \{1, 1, -1, 1\}$, $\sum_i \mu_i = 2$ and $N\{\mu\}=3$.

$\langle N \rangle$ is the average number of oxygenated subunits. It is defined by

$$\langle N \rangle = \sum_{\{\mu\}} P\{\mu\} N\{\mu\}. \tag{4.2.6}$$

Finally, $y = \langle N \rangle / 4$ is the fractional saturation.

It is now possible to introduce the assumptions of the model. These will appear in the relationship between $P\{\mu\}$ and $p(\mu_i)$. Thus, if the subunits are entirely independent of one another,

$$P\{\mu\} = \prod_{i=1}^{4} p(\mu_i), \qquad (4.2.7)$$

which merely states that the probability of a configuration is the product of the probabilities of the individual subunits. If, on the other hand, the subunits interact, (4.2.7) is no longer valid and it becomes necessary to construct a function which reflects the properties of the interaction. We shall assume that

$$P\{\mu\} = \frac{1}{Z} \sum_{i=1}^{4} e^{\mu_i J} e^{U \mu_i \mu_{i+1}} \qquad (4.2.8)$$

with

$$\mu_5 = \mu_1 .$$

U is an interaction parameter; $U = 0$ corresponds to the independent model; $U > 0$ describes a positive or cooperative interaction in the sense that the probability of oxygenation of subunit $i+1$ is increased when subunit i is oxygenated. $U < 0$ is an inhibitory interaction which is of no interest here but may occur in enzymes. An important assumption inherent in (4.2.8) is that only nearest neighbors interact; it is as if the four subunits were arranged in a square pattern and interactions along the sides were permitted but those along the diagonals were prohibited. The quantity Z is a partition function; it is determined from condition (4.2.4), which requires that

$$Z = \sum_{\{\mu\}} \prod_{i=1}^{4} e^{\mu_i J} e^{U \mu_i \mu_{i+1}}, \qquad (4.2.9)$$

or written out in detail,

$$Z = e^{4(U+J)} + 4e^{2J} + 2e^{-4U} + 4e^{-2J} + e^{4(U-J)} + 4. \qquad (4.2.10)$$

The average number of oxygenated subunits, from (4.2.5) and (4.2.6), is

$$\langle N \rangle = \sum_{\{\mu\}} P\{\mu\} \left[2 + \frac{1}{2} \sum_{i=1}^{4} \mu_i \right]$$

$$= \sum_{\{\mu\}} \frac{1}{Z} \prod_{i=1}^{4} e^{\mu_i J} e^{U \mu_i \mu_{i+1}} \left[2 + \frac{1}{2} \sum_{i=1}^{4} \mu_i \right].$$

Since

$$\frac{\partial Z}{\partial J} = \sum_{\{\mu\}} \prod_{i=1}^{4} e^{\mu_i J} e^{U \mu_i \mu_{i+1}} \sum_{i=1}^{4} \mu_i \qquad (4.2.11)$$

we have, from (4.2.9) and (4.2.11)

$$\langle N \rangle = 2 + \frac{1}{2Z} \frac{\partial Z}{\partial J}$$

and

$$y = \frac{\langle N \rangle}{4} = \frac{1}{2} + \frac{1}{8Z} \frac{\partial Z}{\partial J} .$$

With the help of (4.2.10),

$$y = \frac{\alpha[K + (2K + K^2)\alpha + 3K\alpha^2 + \alpha^3]}{1 + 4K\alpha + 2(2K + K^2)\alpha^2 + 4K\alpha^3 + \alpha^4} \tag{4.2.12}$$

where

$$K = e^{-4U}.$$

Eq. (4.2.12) becomes identical with that obtained by KOSHLAND *et al.* (1966) for the "square" case when we set

$$\alpha = K_S K_T [O_2],$$
$$K = K_{AB}^2.$$

When the subunits are independent, $U = 0$, $K = 1$ and (4.2.12) properly reduces to

$$y = \frac{\alpha}{1 + \alpha}, \tag{4.2.13}$$

while at the other extreme, when $U = \infty$, $K = 0$, we obtain

$$y = \frac{\alpha^4}{1 + \alpha^4}, \tag{4.2.14}$$

which corresponds to maximum cooperativity. For hemoglobin, a good fit with experimental equilibrium curves is obtained with $K = 0.11$ or $U = 0.55$ (THOMPSON, 1968).

We see, then, that both models—MWC and KNF—can easily provide a set of parameters consistent with experimental equilibrium curves. However, the predictions from the two models are somewhat different. Whereas the KNF model would predict a sequential change in conformation for each subunit with the possible existence of intermediate structures and a linear relation between the extent of ligand binding and change in conformation, the MWC model predicts a concerted conformational change and no linearity between extent of binding and change in conformation.

4.3 Stereochemical Theory

The stereochemical theory (PERUTZ, 1970, 1972; PERUTZ and TEN EYCK, 1971) provides an explanation of cooperativity and related phenomena such as the Bohr effect in terms of the detailed conformational changes that take place within the hemoglobin molecule when a transition occurs in the state of oxygenation. The underlying concept is that of an interplay between the tertiary structures of the subunits and the quaternary structure of the entire molecule. According to this viewpoint, the quaternary T conformation is regarded as imposing constraints upon the subunits, urging them to adopt or remain in the tertiary t conformation. On the other hand, the quaternary R conformation allows the subunits to adopt the tertiary r conformation. In this sense the T and R conformations are said to be "tense" and "relaxed" respectively.

Suppose, for example, that we have a completely deoxygenated molecule. As we have seen (Section 2.5), the structure would be represented by $[^t\alpha_1\,{}^t\alpha_2\,{}^t\beta_1\,{}^t\beta_2]^T$, which symbolizes the statement that the molecule is in the quaternary T conformation and all the subunits are in the tertiary t conformation. If one of the subunits now makes a transition from t to r, the constraints imposed by the quaternary T form are weakened somewhat and it is easier for another subunit to make the same transition. The constraints imposed by T may now be sufficiently weak for the quaternary structure to go over into the R form. When this occurs the tertiary r form is favored and the remaining t subunits change their conformation to r. The molecule as a whole is now represented by $[^r\alpha_1\,{}^r\alpha_2\,{}^r\beta_1\,{}^r\beta_2]^R$.

We recall that the affinity for oxygen is high in an r and low in a t subunit. Alternatively, it may now be said that since the quaternary R conformation favors the tertiary r conformation, the oxygen affinity is high in R. Conversely, it is low in T. In the stereochemical theory a change in oxygenation in one subunit has no effect on the oxygen affinity of another subunit unless there is a change in the quaternary structure. In other words, the basis for cooperativity is not to be found in any long-range interactions among subunits, but rather in the transition between quaternary R and T conformations.

We shall now summarize the conformational changes that occur during oxygenation as described by the stereochemical theory of PERUTZ (1970). For this purpose it is instructive to refer to Fig. 4.1 which portrays the various stages in the form of a series of schematic diagrams; these, too, are taken from PERUTZ (1970). Fig. 4.1 step 1 shows a completely deoxygenated hemoglobin tetramer containing a molecule of DPG between the two β chains. The tertiary and quaternary structures are in t and T form respectively; hence the hemoglobin molecule in this state is symbolically described by $[^t\alpha_1\,{}^t\alpha_2\,{}^t\beta_1\,{}^t\beta_2]^T$. Let us now imagine that one subunit, say α_1, becomes oxygenated. The following sequence ensues (Fig. 4.1 step 2):

1. In an α chain, the pocket containing the heme is sufficiently ample to allow a ligand like O_2 to enter and bind to iron. Simultaneously with the binding, the iron atom, which in deoxyhemoglobin is situated about 0.75 Å outside the porphyrin plane, moves into the porphyrin plane; the spin changes from high spin $(S=2)$ to low spin $(S=0)$, and the bond between iron and nitrogen $N_{\varepsilon2}$ on the imidazole of the proximal histidine is slightly shortened. When it is recalled that the porphyrin is in contact with about 60 atoms of the globin chain, it is seen that any change in the position of the iron atom and the proximal histidine relative to the porphyrin plane acts as a very effective trigger in starting a sequence of conformational changes. This is a key point in the stereochemical theory.

2. Helix F moves toward helix H, causing the expulsion of tyrosine HC 2 $(140\,\alpha_1)$ which, in deoxyhemoglobin sits between the two helices. The tyrosine pocket shrinks by 1.3 Å so there is no room for tyrosine in oxyhemoglobin.

3. Tyrosine HC 2 $(140\,\alpha_1)$ is the next-to-last residue in the α_1 chain and is therefore attached to the C-terminal residue arginine HC 3 $(141\,\alpha_1)$. Displacement of the tyrosine causes displacement of the normal position of the arginine.

4. In deoxyhemoglobin, arginine HC 3 $(141\,\alpha_1)$ is anchored by two salt bridges to the α_2 chain (Fig. 2.9)—one bridge is to valine NA 2 $(1\,\alpha_2)$ and the other is to aspartate H 9 $(126\,\alpha_2)$. When the arginine is displaced on account of the tyrosine

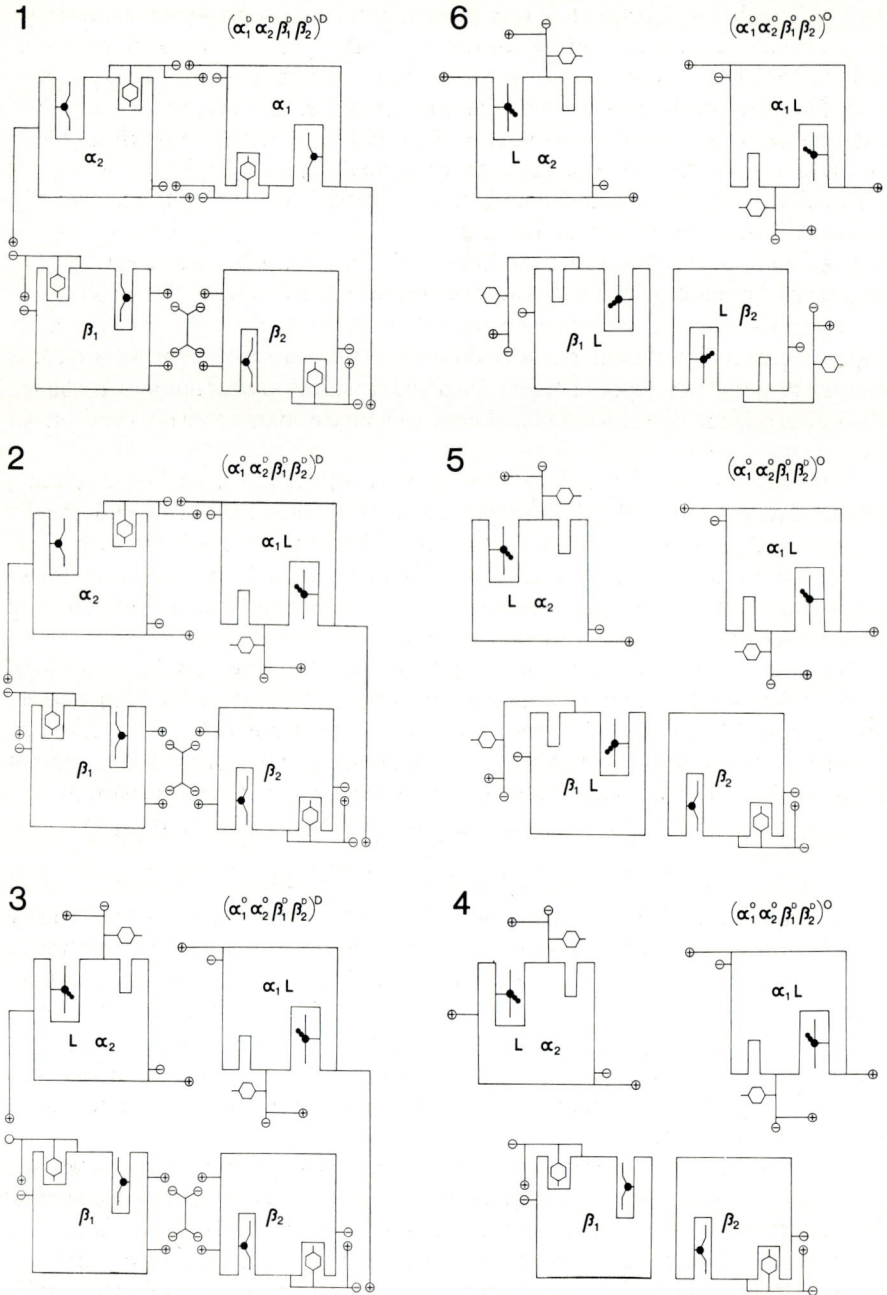

Fig. 4.1. Schematic diagram showing a possible sequence of conformational changes during the oxygenation of hemoglobin (PERUTZ, 1970). Deoxyhemoglobin is shown with one molecule of DPG clamped between the two β chains. The relation between the notation of Perutz and the notation in the text is $\alpha^{0,D} = {}^{r,t}\alpha$, $\beta^{0,D} = {}^{r,t}\beta$ for tertiary conformations and $(\ )^{0,D} = [\ ]^{R,T}$ for quaternary conformations. Recent evidence indicates that in steps 4 and 5 the salt bridges on the β chains should be drawn open (PERUTZ, private communication, 1974).

HC 2 ($140\,\alpha_1$) being expelled from its pocket, the two salt bridges are ruptured. The C-terminal arginine is now free to rotate and the tyrosine has partial freedom.

5. A Bohr proton is released from the α-amino group of valine NA 2 ($1\,\alpha_2$).

6. The α_1 chain is now in the r conformation, i.e. the tertiary structure has made the transition $^t\alpha_1 \to {}^r\alpha_1$. However, the quaternary structure is still in the T conformation. The entire structure is described by $[^r\alpha_1\,^t\alpha_2\,^t\beta_1\,^t\beta_2]^T$.

A β chain goes through a similar but not identical sequence. The steps for β_1, say, are as follows (Fig. 4.1 step 5):

1. In contrast with the situation in an α chain, there is not sufficient room in the pocket containing the heme to accommodate a ligand. Hence the pocket must first open with the help of energy derived from thermal vibrations. When an oxygen molecule finally enters, the iron atom $Fe\,\beta_1$ switches from its displaced position in deoxyhemoglobin to the in-plane position and undergoes a change in spin state from $S=2$ to $S=0$. These events are identical with those in an α chain.

2. Helix F moves toward helix H, thereby constricting the pocket containing tyrosing HC 2 ($145\,\beta_1$). As a consequence the tyrosine is expelled and the C-terminal residue histidine HC 3 ($146\,\beta_1$) attached to the tyrosine is displaced.

3. In deoxyhemoglobin, histidine HC 3 ($146\,\beta_1$) is ionically bonded to aspartate FG 1 ($94\,\beta_1$) (Fig. 2.9). This salt bridge is now ruptured and the histidine is free to rotate and the tyrosine attached to it is partially free.

Thus the transitions of α and β subunits from t to r loosen up the quaternary structure by successively rupturing salt bridges until the strains occasioned by some subunits' being in r while the quaternary structure is in T are sufficient to produce the transition T→R. This is shown as occurring between steps 3 and 4 of Fig. 4.1. The entire sequence of steps 1 to 6 corresponds to the transitions

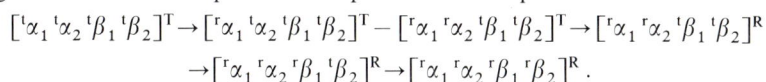

$$[^t\alpha_1\,^t\alpha_2\,^t\beta_1\,^t\beta_2]^T \to [^r\alpha_1\,^t\alpha_2\,^t\beta_1\,^t\beta_2]^T - [^r\alpha_1\,^r\alpha_2\,^t\beta_1\,^t\beta_2]^T \to [^r\alpha_1\,^r\alpha_2\,^t\beta_1\,^t\beta_2]^R$$
$$\to [^r\alpha_1\,^r\alpha_2\,^r\beta_1\,^t\beta_2]^R \to [^r\alpha_1\,^r\alpha_2\,^r\beta_1\,^r\beta_2]^R \ .$$

The transitions, of course, need not occur in exactly this sequence; it is merely one of several plausible sequences consistent with the overall picture, though there is growing evidence (LINDSTROM and HO, 1972) that the binding of oxygen is indeed sequential; α subunits react first, followed by the β subunits. The main point is that cooperativity, whereby the binding or release of oxygen from one subunit appears to have an effect on other subunits, is inextricably linked with a change in quaternary conformation. The subunits themselves exert no direct influence on one another.

The stereochemical theory provides a qualitative picture of cooperativity. How do other features of the oxygenation process fit in with this viewpoint? The first and most important is the alkaline (physiological) Bohr effect. Any explanation of this effect presupposes the existence of residues whose protons are more tightly bound in deoxyhemoglobin than in oxyhemoglobin. An equivalent statement is that for such a residue

$$pK_{oxy} < pK_{deoxy},$$

or that the residue is more acidic in oxyhemoglobin and hence releases protons more readily. Two main sources for this effect have been identified:

1. The imidazole groups of the two C-terminal histidines HC 3 (146 β). In deoxyhemoglobin each of these groups is linked by a salt bridge to the β-carboxyl of aspartate FG 1 (94 β). In oxyhemoglobin these salt bridges are broken and the histidines are free to rotate. This means that in deoxyhemoglobin the proton in imidazole is bound more securely due to interaction with the negative charge of carboxyl in aspartate. Hence the pK of the imidazole is lowered upon oxygenation; this accounts for about half of the Bohr effect.

2. The α-amino groups in valines NA 2 (1 α), each of which is linked in deoxyhemoglobin to the α-carboxyl of arginine HC 3 (141 α) of the partner chain. As before, the salt bridges are broken upon oxygenation and the result is a lowered pK for the α-amino group. About one fourth of the Bohr effect is ascribed to these groups.

The rest of the Bohr effect is attributed to various other groups, such as the imidazole group of histidine, H 5 (122 α), which comes close to a negatively charged carboxyl group in deoxyhemoglobin, whereas in oxyhemoglobin it approaches a positively charged guanidinium group.

The explanation of the Bohr effect on this basis automatically accounts for the observed proportionality between the amount of oxygen taken up and the number of protons released. What is perhaps even more important is the intimate connection between the cooperative characteristics and the Bohr effect that emerges from the stereochemical theory. It is clear that anything that will impair the Bohr effect will also reduce the cooperative interaction and vice versa. Hence a system like myoglobin, whose equilibrium curve is hyperbolic, is not subject to a Bohr effect.

There are a number of additional experimental observations which lend support to the stereochemical theory. Among these are the following:

1. It is possible to remove the C-terminal residues arginine HC 3 (141 α) and histidine HC 3 (146 β). The effect is to reduce the Hill constant from its normal value of about 2.8 to close to unity and to increase the oxygen affinity. At the same time the Bohr effect disappears. At first sight this is rather strange, since the C-terminal residues have nothing to do with the heme. However, it is quite clear from the stereochemical picture. The C-terminal residues form salt bridges in deoxyhemoglobin; if these residues are removed, the salt bridges are destroyed and the T conformation cannot be established. Since the molecule nevertheless binds oxygen reversibly, the reaction takes place between the two forms

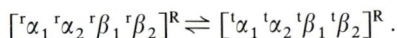

$$[^r\alpha_1{}^r\alpha_2{}^r\beta_1{}^r\beta_2]^R \rightleftharpoons [^t\alpha_1{}^t\alpha_2{}^t\beta_1{}^t\beta_2]^R .$$

The form on the right is a very strange one in that it consists of deoxygenated subunits in quaternary R conformation, the latter normally being associated with oxyhemoglobin. This is a striking example of the importance of the quaternary conformation in the oxygenation process.

2. The reagent BME (bis-N-maleimido methyl ether) locks hemoglobin into the R conformation. It accomplishes this by linking cysteine F 9 (93 β) to histidine FG 4 (97 β) on the same β chain. With BME present, hemoglobin can still bind oxygen reversibly but, as in the previous case, the affinity for oxygen is increased, the equilibrium curve is hyperbolic ($n=1$) and there is no Bohr effect. The

significance of this observation is again to demonstrate the intimate relationship between cooperativity and the Bohr effect on the one hand and quaternary conformational changes on the other: When anything interferes with the quaternary conformational changes both cooperativity and the Bohr effect are lost.

3. As we have noted, DPG reduces the affinity of hemoglobin for oxygen and produces a shift in the equilibrium curve in the direction of higher oxygen pressures. One mole of DPG binds strongly to one mole of deoxyhemoglobin, but very weakly, if at all, to oxyhemoglobin. The effect of DPG is to lock hemoglobin into the T form, so that in order to bind oxygen, the DPG molecule has to be displaced or expelled. Other evidence indicates that DPG interacts only with β chains and probably occupies a position along the two-fold axis where it can crosslink the two β chains by forming additional salt bridges (Fig. 4.1). From the stereochemical viewpoint, DPG therefore inhibits the conformational transition T→R. This then biases the equilibrium in favor of deoxyhemoglobin, which is, of course, equivalent to reducing the oxygen affinity.

4. Magnetic resonance experiments employing electronic spin labels and those based on proton resonances are capable of probing localized regions of the molecule. The results obtained by these methods (described in the next section) are entirely consistent with the stereochemical viewpoint.

5. There has been much discussion on the identity of the fundamental cooperative unit—whether it is an $\alpha\beta$ dimer or the complete tetramer. The stereochemical theory, with its emphasis on the quaternary conformations, comes out in favor of the tetramer (PERUTZ, 1970). This hypothesis is supported by such observations as a) the lack of any significant dependence of cooperativity on the concentration of hemoglobin, b) the fact that the Hill constant for hemoglobin is greater than 2, c) the reluctance of deoxyhemoglobin to dissociate into dimers, contrasted with oxyhemoglobin's tendency to dissociation, and d) the absence of cooperativity in the oxygenation of $\alpha_1\beta_1$ dimers. Taken in conjunction with the unified picture of a wide range of experimental information provided by the stereochemical theory, this evidence must lend considerable weight to the tetrameric hypothesis.

4.4 Magnetic Resonance

Several kinds of magnetic resonance methods have been applied to hemoglobin: electron spin resonance (ESR or EPR) associated with a spin label attached to the molecule, nuclear magnetic resonance (NMR) associated with protons that are part of the molecule, and ESR associated with iron in a paramagnetic state. In this section we discuss the first two methods, since the results that have been obtained are relevant to the cooperative mechanism; the third will be treated in Chapter VI, which also contains some of the basic theory pertaining to magnetic resonance.

The spin-label technique is one of a class of methods which employ microprobes attached to a macromolecule to sample the local environment. In the method employed by MCCONNELL and his colleagues (MCCONNELL and MCFARLAND, 1970; MCCONNELL, 1971; OGATA and MCCONNELL, 1971, 1972), the spin label consists of a nitroxide radical (Fig. 4.2), which is attached to some specific site on the hemoglobin molecule. Radicals of this type contain an electron with an unpaired spin ($S=1/2$) in the $2p\pi$ orbital of nitrogen. Such radicals

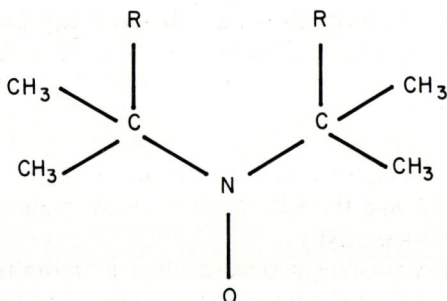

Fig. 4.2. Nitroxide radical. The attachment of the radical to a macromolecule is accomplished by means of the reactive groups R

are therefore paramagnetic and are capable of producing an ESR (electron spin resonance) spectrum. In solution, at room temperature, the radicals rotate at a rate sufficiently rapid to average out all existing anisotropies. The spectrum then consists of three lines as a result of the isotropic hyperfine interaction between the unpaired electron and the nitrogen nucleus which has a spin of 1. If the motion of the radical is hindered in any way, e.g. by attachment to a macromolecule, the anisotropies may no longer average zero. In this case the three-line spectrum is subject to changes varying in their degree of complication. The ESR spectrum is therefore strongly influenced by the motion of the radical.

A spin label attached to a macromolecule is subject to two kinds of motion. One kind is the rotational diffusion of the large molecule; this motion is slow and does not average out anisotropies. The second is the rotation of the label relative to the macromolecule, and this motion is determined almost entirely by the local conformation. At one extreme the label may be completely free to rotate, while at the opposite extreme the conformation of the macromolecule may be such as to totally immobilize the label. The alteration in the three-line ESR spectrum of the spin label when it is attached to a macromolecule can therefore yield information on the local conformation in the vicinity of the label. Labels I, II, and III are among those that have been used in experiments on hemoglobin.

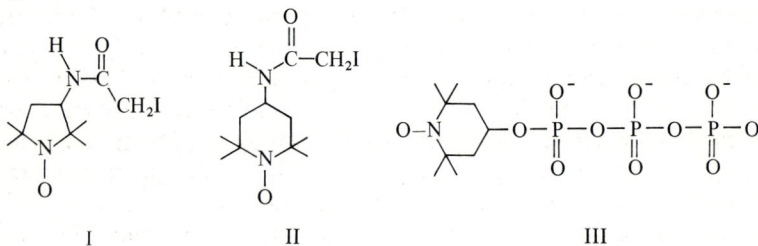

I   II   III

Labels I and II were covalently bonded to the reactive sulphydryl group in cysteine F 9 (93 β); label III, in all likelihood, occupied a site similar to that of DPG, i.e. between the two β subunits.

We shall now summarize the principal results obtained from spin label experiments and their interpretation as to the mode of action of hemoglobin. It will be convenient to discuss labels I and II separately from label III since, as we have seen, the binding sites in the two cases are quite different.

Labels I and II

1. The affinity of hemoglobin for oxygen with the label attached is increased by a factor of about 10, and the Hill constant drops to about 2.3 indicating that there is some loss in cooperativity.

2. The ESR spectrum changes when oxygen is bound to deoxyhemoglobin, and the fractional change in the signal is proportional to the amount of oxygen that is bound. From the viewpoint of the stereochemical theory the spin label is in such a position that in oxyhemoglobin it may enter the pocket vacated by the penultimate tyrosine HC 2 (145 β). In this case the label is essentially immobilized. In deoxyhemoglobin, the pocket is occupied by tyrosine, so the spin label is free. Since β chains have open pockets only when oxygenated, it is expected that there will be a proportionality between the change in the signal and the amount of oxygen bound to β chains. Since the change in the signal is taken as a measure of the conformational change in the region of the label, a linear relation can be said to exist between the conformational change in the vicinity of cysteine F 9 (93 β) and heme oxygenation.

3. The reactivity of the SH group in cysteine F 9 (93 β) to which spin labels are attached is much lower in deoxyhemoglobin than in oxyhemoglobin. The reason is that histidine HC 3 (146 β) is fixed in position by the salt bridge with aspartate FG 1 (94 β) in deoxyhemoglobin. In this fixed position the histidine blocks access to the cysteine. In oxyhemoglobin the histidine is free and does not block the path to the SH group. Again the reactivity must be proportional to the amount of oxygen that is bound.

4. An important aspect of spin label experiments has to do with the presence or absence of isosbestic points—a term borrowed from absorption spectroscopy. For ESR experiments, an isosbestic point is a value of the magnetic field at which the spectra of two species, say A and B, cross. In other words, when A and B are mixed and a series of spectra are obtained with different concentrations of A and B but keeping the total concentration fixed, the signal at an isosbestic point will remain unchanged. The importance of such points is that their presence is an indication that two, and only two, species contribute to the spectra. In the hemoglobin experiments, a slight deviation from isosbesty as a function of oxygenation was observed. This then suggests that there are more than two conformations in the vicinity of the label. A possible interpretation on the basis of the stereochemical theory is that in addition to the fully oxygenated $[^r\alpha_1{}^r\alpha_2{}^r\beta_1{}^r\beta_2]^R$ and the deoxygenated $[^t\alpha_1{}^t\alpha_2{}^t\beta_1{}^t\beta_2]^T$ conformations there must also be one or more intermediate conformations, such as $[^r\alpha_1{}^r\alpha_2{}^t\beta_1{}^t\beta_2]^R$. In this case the β subunits may be expected to be under strain since their tertiary

structures are in the t form, whereas the quaternary structure has already flipped to the R form.

5. Experiments were conducted with hybrid hemoglobins such as $\alpha_2(Fe^{3+}CN)\beta_2$ and $\alpha_2\beta_2(Fe^{3+}CN)$. In the former the two α chains are in the ferric state and are liganded with CN^- while the two β chains are in the ferrous state and may be oxygenated or not. In the second variety the role of the α and β chains is reversed, but in both varieties, it must be remembered, the spin labels are on the β chains only. The results of studying the ESR spectra of such hybrids as a function of oxygenation indicate that the label senses oxygenation on the β chains but responds only very weakly when the α chains are oxygenated. This suggests that oxygenation in a particular chain produces a change in tertiary structure of that chain but effects on neighboring chains are greatly reduced.

Label III

1. The effects of the triphosphate label are similar to those of DPG (Section 3.3). The label binds preferentially to deoxyhemoglobin; the oxygen affinity is reduced but the cooperative properties remain unaltered.

2. The ESR spectra of the label change as a function of oxygen (or CO) saturation; isosbestic points have been observed.

3. When used with the hybrid hemoglobins, the triphosphate label binds more strongly to $\alpha_2(Fe^{3+}CN)\beta_2$ than to $\alpha_2\beta_2(Fe^{3+}CN)$. These experiments, as well as experiments with certain mutant varieties of hemoglobin, have indicated quite conclusively that α and β subunits are not equivalent.

Nuclear magnetic resonance (NMR) provides another method of probing local conformational changes (WUTHRICH, 1970; OGAWA *et al.*, 1972). In this case the macromolecule's own protons constitute the probes, by virtue of each proton possessing a magnetic moment. As with the spin label method, observations can be made at various temperatures, in solution or in single crystals, but this method differs from the spin label method in that it is not necessary to attach any external groups to the macromolecule. At first sight it might appear unlikely that an NMR spectrum of a molecule as large as hemoglobin would yield much information, since there are some 4000 protons and the resonances are broadened by the slow rotation of the molecule. This is true of most of the protons, but not all of them. In particular, the protons associated with the heme may have resonances located away from the rest.

In ferrihemoglobin, it is possible for the unpaired electrons in Fe, which are the source of the molecule's paramagnetism, to interact with the protons situated near the periphery of the porphyrin ring. Such hyperfine interactions result in shifts of the proton resonances, and if these shifts are large in comparison to the line widths, it is then possible to extract useful information from the NMR spectra. A necessary condition before the paramagnetic shifts can be large is a short relaxation time for the electronic spins (WUTHRICH, 1970). For this purpose, low-spin ($S=1/2$) ferrihemoglobin (e.g. HbCN) is preferable to the high-spin form because of the presence of spin orbit coupling which helps to reduce the relaxation time (see Chapter V and VIII). Two contributions to the paramagnetically shifted resonances may be distinguished.

1. Unpaired electron spin density is transferred from the iron atom into the π-orbital system of the porphyrin from which it is further transferred to the peripheral protons. In effect, the electronic spin of the iron becomes delocalized and produces a magnetic field at the positions of the protons. This then is the contact hyperfine interaction which shifts the proton resonances; it is isotropic and the shifts are inversely proportional to the absolute temperature.

2. Another isotropic interaction which contributes to the paramagnetic shifts in the proton resonances is known as the pseudo-contact interaction. For this to exist the paramagnetism of the molecule must be characterized by an anisotropic g tensor, i.e. the magnetic moment depends on the direction of the magnetic field relative to the molecular axes. When one considers the dipolar interaction between the electronic spins (mainly on the iron atom) and the proton spins, taking into account the anisotropic g tensor, and the interaction is averaged over all orientations of the molecule (as in solution), the pseudo-contact interaction is obtained. The interaction depends on the positions of the protons relative to the iron and varies with distance as $1/r^3$. Since delocalization of electronic spins is not involved, the pseudo-contact interaction is independent of the specifics of the bonding arrangement.

A magnetic field applied to a closed conjugated system like porphyrin (or an aromatic amino acid) produces a Larmor precession in the π-electron system. This is usually known as a ring current. The resulting magnetic field also shifts the proton resonances. However, in the NMR investigations of hemoglobin these diamagnetic shifts were only of minor importance.

As a result of these interactions, the protons associated with the heme are shifted to higher and lower fields so that in myoglobin it has been possible to assign resonances to specific groups of the heme. In hemoglobin, because of its larger size, the resonances are broader; the analysis of the spectrum is therefore less detailed. Even in hemoglobin, however, when methods developed by SHULMAN and his colleagues are used (OGAWA et al., 1972; OGAWA et al., 1972a, OGAWA and SHULMAN, 1972), these resonances are sufficiently distinct to monitor changes that may occur in the vicinity of the heme. Most of the work was done with ferricyanide complexes in various forms—isolated chains, HbCN and the mixed hybrids $\alpha_2\beta_2(Fe^{3+}CN)$ and $\alpha_2(Fe^{3+}CN)\beta_2$. The NMR signal, it must be remembered, refers only to the paramagnetically shifted resonances and is associated entirely with the ferricyanide chains.

The most revealing experiments with implications for the mechanism of cooperativity were those performed with the mixed hybrids. In $\alpha_2(Fe^{3+}CN)\beta_2$, in which the α subunits are unliganded, two kinds of NMR spectra were observed, depending on whether DPG had been added or not. This was taken as an indication that the hybrid can reside in either of two different structures. Further, the NMR spectrum of $\alpha_2(Fe^{3+}CN)\beta_2$ without DPG was very similar to the spectrum of the oxygenated form $[\alpha_2(Fe^{3+}CN)\beta_2(O_2)_2]$. The latter is presumed to be in the quaternary R conformation. Therefore, on the assumption that spectral changes correspond to changes in quaternary conformation, it was concluded that the quaternary R conformation is favored by $\alpha_2(Fe^{3+}CN)\beta_2$ without DPG. On the other hand, since DPG is known to bind preferentially to deoxyhemoglobin, which is in the T conformation, the altered spectrum of

$\alpha_2(Fe^{3+}CN)\beta_2$ on addition of DPG (or other phosphates) meant that the quaternary conformation had switched from R to T. The general conclusion was that the mixed hybrid in solution can exist in either the R or the T quaternary conformation, that the two conformations are in equilibrium and that the equilibrium can be shifted from one conformation to the other. By implication, this means that in partially oxygenated hemoglobin in which the α subunits are oxygenated but not the β subunits, there is an equilibrium between the two forms $[^r\alpha_1{}^r\alpha_2{}^l\beta_1{}^l\beta_2]^R$ and $[^r\alpha_1{}^r\alpha_2{}^l\beta_1{}^l\beta_2]^T$.

The results of experiments with $\alpha_2\beta_2(Fe^{3+}CN)$ were similar, except that it was more difficult to perform the switch between the R and T conformations, which provides additional evidence for the non-equivalence of α and β subunits.

Finally, the observation that hybrids in the R conformation combine with CO at a much faster rate than those in the T conformation was interpreted as an indication that a quaternary change is a necessary requirement for cooperativity.

4.5 Discussion

The central fact that is consistent with all experiments performed with hemoglobin so far is that cooperativity cannot occur without concomitant changes in the quaternary conformation. The problem then, as phrased by HOPFIELD (1973), is to understand how "the protein modulates the binding energy" of the heme so that, "the fourth oxygen molecule bound has a free energy of binding which is 3.6 kcal/mole greater than the free energy of binding of the first oxygen molecule".

From the standpoint of thermodynamics, the MWC and KNF models, with suitable parametrization, are both capable of describing the sigmoidal shape of the oxygen equilibrium curve to within experimental accuracy. Hence, on this basis alone both models have equal validity. However, the realization of the importance of the quaternary conformation lent support to the MWC model, which assumes that there is an equilibrium between two structures—these could be interpreted as the quaternary structures—whose affinities for oxygen are very different. The advent of the NMR data, which strongly suggested that hemoglobin can exist in two different quaternary conformations and yet maintain the same degree of oxygenation, finally tipped the weight of experimental evidence in favor of the MWC model. As a final step, existing kinetic data were examined from the standpoint of the MWC model (HOPFIELD et al., 1971) and it was found that it was indeed possible to derive a set of first-order kinetic and equilibrium constants consistent with all known kinetic binding data on normal and mutant hemoglobins.

However, the MWC model, it must be remembered, does not distinguish between α and β subunits, and this is contrary to evidence from various sources (X-ray structure, spin labels, NMR). Still, it could be argued that the non-equivalence of the subunits might not be so important, since there were after all no serious quantitative discrepancies between the model and experimental data. This viewpoint appears not to be tenable any longer in view of recent experiments by GIBSON (1973), who observed substantial differences in the kinetic binding constants of α and β chains. He concludes that "the Monod-Wyman-Changeux model is quite unsuited to represent the kinetics of the oxygen-hemoglobin reaction".

A model which is presumably not open to objections of this kind is one developed by OGATA and McCONNELL (1971, 1972). The basic features of the MWC model are retained, but without the assumption of chain equivalence. In place of the three parameters L, C, α (Section 4.1) the extended model contains five parameters, L, C_α, C_β, α, β (or L, k_R^α, k_R^β, k_T^α, k_T^β) which have been fitted satisfactorily to data on oxygen dissociation, spin labels and NMR for several kinds of hemoglobin.

Thermodynamic models provide quantitative descriptions but do not say anything specific about molecular mechanisms. On the other hand, the molecular mechanism of PERUTZ (1970) is largely qualitative. To bridge this gap, SZABO and KARPLUS (1972) developed a model which conforms to the known structure of hemoglobin. It assumes two quaternary conformations (R and T) and two tertiary conformations for each subunit—one corresponding to the oxygenated form (r) and the other to the deoxygenated form (t). It is also assumed, with PERUTZ, that the interchain salt bridges provide the coupling between the tertiary and quaternary conformations. The model may therefore be regarded as the thermodynamic counterpart to the Perutz mechanism. Whether in fact the salt bridges serve to couple the tertiary and quaternary structures, or in thermodynamic terms, whether the difference in free energy between the two quaternary conformations is localized in the interchain salt bridges, appears to be open to question. In the view of OGAWA and SHULMAN (1972) and HOPFIELD (1973) the NMR data suggest that the free energy is delocalized, that is, it is spread out over many bonds.

Chapter V

Electronic States of Iron

The description of the electronic states of iron in hemoglobin has been approached through crystal field theory and molecular orbital theory, and by a combination of the two, which is known as ligand field theory. Each approach provides certain insights, though none is entirely satisfactory. In all cases, however, symmetry is of paramount importance. We shall therefore devote this chapter to a summary of the results pertaining to Fe^{2+} and Fe^{3+} which are largely consequences of the symmetry of the environment in which the ion is immersed. A natural starting point is the free ion whose symmetry is that of the full rotation group.

5.1 Free Ions

The electronic configurations of Fe^{3+} and Fe^{2+}, outside of closed shells, are $(3d)^5$ and $(3d)^6$ respectively. As a result of Coulomb interactions, each configuration gives rise to a set of terms; those that satisfy the Pauli principle are listed in Table 5.1. The superscript on the left is the multiplicity $(2S+1)$ and the subscript is the seniority number $(v)^5$; thus ^4_5D means $L=2, S=\frac{3}{2}, v=5$. Energies to first order are expressed in terms of Racah coefficients which are defined for d electrons by

$$A = F^{(0)} - \tfrac{49}{441} F^{(4)} = F_0 - 49 F_4 ,$$
$$B = \tfrac{1}{49} F^{(2)} - \tfrac{5}{441} F^{(4)} = F_2 - 5 F_4 ,$$
$$C = \tfrac{35}{441} F^{(4)} = 35 F_4 , \tag{5.1.1}$$

$$F^{(k)} = e^2 \int_0^\infty \int_0^\infty \frac{r_<^k}{r_>^{k+1}} [R_{nl}(r_1) R_{nl}(r_2)]^2 dr_1 dr_2 ,$$

where $R_{nl}(r)$ is the radial part of the one-electron wave function

$$\psi_{nlm}(r, \theta, \varphi) = \frac{1}{r} R_{nl}(r) Y_{lm}(\theta, \varphi) . \tag{5.1.2}$$

---

[5] For the d^n configuration several multiplets occur with the same value of L and S. Thus, for d^5 (Table 5.1), ^2G occurs twice, ^2F twice, and ^2D three times. The seniority number, v, is an additional quantum number which serves to distinguish such multiplets (see, for example, SLATER, 1960).

Terms like ^2_5D and ^2_1D, which are alike except for seniority number, may interact and give rise to nonvanishing off-diagonal matrix elements of the Coulomb operator. Table 5.1 lists the eigenvalues of the corresponding 2×2 matrices in such cases. The seniority number appears only in special situations; we shall therefore not retain reference to it except as needed. For Fe^{3+}, $B = 1015 \text{ cm}^{-1}$, $C = 4800 \text{ cm}^{-1}$, and for Fe^{2+}, $B = 917 \text{ cm}^{-1}$, $C = 4040 \text{ cm}^{-1}$ (KOTANI, 1968);

Table 5.1. *Terms arising from d^5 and d^6 electronic configurations. A, B and C are Racah coefficients*

	Term	Energy
d^5	^6_5S	$10A - 35B$
	^4_5G	$10A - 25B + 5C$
	^4_3F	$10A - 13B + 7C$
	^4_5D	$10A - 18B + 5C$
	^4_3P	$10A - 28B + 7C$
	^2_5I	$10A - 24B + 8C$
	^2_3H	$10A - 22B + 10C$
	^2_5G	$10A - 13B + 8C$
	^2_3G	$10A + 3B + 10C$
	^2_5F	$10A - 9B + 8C$
	^2_3F	$10A - 25B + 10C$
	^2_3D	$10A - 4B + 10C$
	$^2_5D, {}^2_1D$	$10A - 3B + 11C \pm 3(57B^2 + 2BC + C^2)^{\frac{1}{2}}$
	^2_3P	$10A + 20B + 10C$
	^2_5S	$10A - 3B + 8C$
d^6	^5_4D	$6A - 21B$
	^3_4H	$6A - 17B + 4C$
	^3_4G	$6A - 12B + 4C$
	$^3_4F, {}^3_2F$	$6A - 5B + 5\frac{1}{2}C \pm \frac{3}{2}(68B^2 + 4BC + C^2)^{\frac{1}{2}}$
	^3_4D	$6A - 5B + 4C$
	$^3_4P, {}^3_2P$	$6A - 5B + 5\frac{1}{2}C \pm \frac{1}{2}(912B^2 - 24BC + 9C^2)^{\frac{1}{2}}$
	^1_4I	$6A - 15B + 6C$
	$^1_4G, {}^1_2G$	$6A - 5B + 7\frac{1}{2}C \pm \frac{1}{2}(708B^2 - 12BC + 9C^2)^{\frac{1}{2}}$
	^1_4F	$6A + 6C$
	$^1_4D, {}^1_2D$	$6A + 9B + 7\frac{1}{2}C \pm \frac{3}{2}(144B^2 + 8BC + C^2)^{\frac{1}{2}}$
	$^1_4S, {}^1_0S$	$6A + 10B + 10C \pm 2(193B^2 + 8BC + 4C^2)^{\frac{1}{2}}$

A need not be specified if only relative energies are of interest. A particular term arising from an electronic configuration l^n may be regarded as a daughter of various parent terms associated with the configuration l^{n-1}. As a simple example, the ^2D term of p^3 can be considered as the daughter of ^3P and ^1D belonging to p^2 since a third p electron can be coupled either to ^3P or to ^1D to produce ^2D. Similarly, the parents of ^4P in d^5 are the terms ^5D, ^3_4F, ^3_2F, ^3D, ^3_4P, ^3_2P in d^4; ^6S in d^5 has only one parent in d^4, namely ^5D. The practical advantage of this point of view is that a knowledge of the parent wave functions leads to a formulation of the daughter wave function,

$$|l^n S L\rangle = \sum_{S'L'} |l^{n-1}(S'\,L')l S L\rangle \langle l^{n-1}(S'\,L')l S L| \} l^n S L\rangle . \qquad (5.1.3)$$

The coefficients $\langle l^{n-1}(S'L')lSL|\} l^nSL\rangle$ are known as fractional parentage coefficients (cfp).

Electronic terms will be further affected by spin-orbit coupling, represented by the operator

$$\mathcal{H}_s = \sum_i \zeta(r_i)\mathbf{l}_i \cdot \mathbf{s}_i \tag{5.1.4}$$

where the summation is taken over all the electrons in the configuration (outside of closed shells). Interactions may occur within a particular term or between terms. Most often it is necessary to evaluate matrix elements in an $|SLJM_J\rangle$ basis set; since $\mathcal{H}_s$ is expressed in terms of one-electron operators it would, in principle, be necessary to expand $|SLJM_J\rangle$ into products of one-electron states and to calculate the one-electron matrix elements. Needless to say, this procedure would be rather tedious; much more elegant methods have been developed by RACAH and are described in various books, including SLATER (1960), JUDD (1963), and WATANABE (1966). A convenient expression with accompanying tables is given by SLATER; for equivalent electrons

$$\langle SLJM_J|\mathcal{H}_s|S'L'J'M_J'\rangle = \delta(J,J')\delta(M_J,M_J')\zeta_{nl}(-1)^{L+S'+J}[l(l+1)(2l+1)]^{1/2}$$
$$\times (SL\|V''\|S'L')\begin{Bmatrix} S & L & J \\ L' & S' & 1 \end{Bmatrix} \tag{5.1.5}$$

in which $(SL\|V''\|S'L')$ is a reduced matrix element; the quantity in curly brackets is a 6-j symbol (ROTENBERG et al., 1959), which is closely related to Racah's W-coefficient:

$$\begin{Bmatrix} S & L & J \\ L' & S' & 1 \end{Bmatrix} = (-1)^{S+L+S'+L'}W(SLS'L';J1). \tag{5.1.6}$$

Eq. (5.1.5) contains certain selection rules:

$$\begin{aligned} \Delta J &= 0, \\ \Delta M_J &= 0, \\ \Delta S &= 0, \pm 1 \quad \text{but not } 0 \to 0, \\ \Delta L &= 0, \pm 1 \quad \text{but not } 0 \to 0. \end{aligned} \tag{5.1.7}$$

The first two are stated explicitly; the last two are contained in the properties of the 6-j symbol.

Let us now investigate the effect of spin-orbit coupling on the ^6S ground term of d^5. In the first place there can be no spin-orbit coupling within the ^6S term alone. As a consequence of the selection rules (5.1.7), ^6S interacts only with ^4P, which lies some 41000 cm^{-1} higher. All other matrix elements of $\mathcal{H}_s$ involving the ground term must vanish.

For d^5 and $S=\frac{5}{2}$, $L=0$, $S'=\frac{3}{2}$, $L'=1$, SLATER's tables give

$$(\tfrac{5}{2}0\|V''\|\tfrac{3}{2}1) = (^6S\|V''\|^4P) = \sqrt{3}.$$

The 6-j symbol, with $J=\frac{5}{2}$, has the value $-\sqrt{2}/6$. We therefore have

$$\langle d^{5\,6}S_{\frac{5}{2}}|\mathcal{H}_s|d^{5\,4}P_{\frac{5}{2}}\rangle = \sqrt{5}\,\zeta_{nl} \tag{5.1.8}$$

where ζ_{nl} is known as the spin-orbit coupling parameter and is defined by the radial integral

$$\zeta_{nl} = \int [R_{nl}(r)]^2 \zeta(r) dr . \tag{5.1.9}$$

Since we shall only be concerned with $3d$ electors $(n=3, l=2)$, the subscripts on ζ_{nl} are redundant and we will write $\zeta_{nl}=\zeta$. For Fe^{3+}, ζ is 435 cm^{-1}.

Expression (5.1.5) can also be used to calculate the spin-orbit coupling within the ^4P term of d^5, but this is superfluous because there is no splitting within a term arising from a half-filled shell.

In summary, the matrix of $\mathscr{H}_s$ within the set of terms consisting of ^6S and ^4P is

$\mathscr{H}_s$	^6S	^4P
^6S	0	$-\sqrt{5}\zeta$
^4P	$-\sqrt{5}\zeta$	$0.$

From Table 5.1, to second order in ζ,

$$E(^6S) = 10\,A - 35\,B - \frac{5\zeta^2}{7(B+C)} ,$$

$$|^6S\rangle' = |^6S\rangle - \frac{\sqrt{5}\zeta}{7(B+C)}|^4P\rangle \tag{5.1.10}$$

where $|^6S\rangle'$ is the ground state corrected to first order for spin-orbit coupling.

5.2 Cubic Symmetry

In all hemoglobin derivatives the iron atom is coordinated to six ligands, except for deoxyhemoglobin in which the iron is 5-coordinated. To a first approximation we may idealize the environment of the iron atom to an octahedral arrangement of identical ligands, that is, one ligand at each of the positions $x = \pm a$, $y = \pm a$, $z = \pm a$. Ligands disposed in this fashion are said to produce a symmetrical environment whose symmetry elements are those contained in the cubic group O_h. Ultimately, it will be necessary to take departures from the ideal octahedral arrangement into account and have recourse to lower symmetry groups.

5.2.1 Symmetry Elements

The entire set of covering operations of the cube, i.e. the set of proper and improper rotations which send a cube into itself, constitute the elements of the group O_h. The proper rotations by themselves form a subgroup O; hence the group O_h may be regarded as the direct product of O and C_i where C_i is the two-element group consisting of the identity and inversion operators. The elements of O, including those associated with the spinor or double group, are listed in Table 5.2.

Although we have spoken of the elements of the cubic group as covering operations, which brings to mind the picture of an object being rotated, an equally valid interpretation is to regard the elements as coordinate transforma-

Table 5.2. *Symmetry elements and characters of the cubic group* O, *including the double (spinor) group*

O		E	$\bar{E}$	$8C_3$	$8\bar{C}_3$	$3C_2$ $3\bar{C}_2$	$6C_4$	$6\bar{C}_4$	$6C'_2$ $6\bar{C}'_2$
A_1	Γ_1	1	1	1	1	1	1	1	1
A_2	Γ_2	1	1	1	1	1	-1	-1	-1
E	Γ_3	2	2	-1	-1	2	0	0	0
T_1	Γ_4	3	3	0	0	-1	1	1	-1
T_2	Γ_5	3	3	0	0	-1	-1	-1	1
E'	Γ_6	2	-2	1	-1	0	$\sqrt{2}$	$-\sqrt{2}$	0
E''	Γ_7	2	-2	1	-1	0	$-\sqrt{2}$	$\sqrt{2}$	0
U'	Γ_8	4	-4	-1	1	0	0	0	0

Definitions (refer to Fig. 5.1)

E = identity operation
$\bar{E}$ = rotation through an angle of 2π about an arbitrary axis
C_3 = a rotation of $\pm\dfrac{2\pi}{3}$ about any one of the 4 body diagonals such as AB
C_2 = a rotation of π about any one of the 3 coordinate axes
C_4 = a rotation of $\pm\dfrac{\pi}{2}$ about any one of the 3 coordinate axes
C'_2 = a rotation of π about any one of 6 axes which bisect opposite sides, such as CD.
A bar over an element indicates multiplication by $\bar{E}$ e.g. $\bar{C}_4 = C_4\bar{E}$.

tions. There is no particular advantage to one interpretation or the other; the important point is to keep them distinct and separate to avoid the hopeless confusion which would result from mixing the two interpretations. We shall regard the elements as coordinate transformations. To be specific, any element R such as C_2, C_3, etc., will be understood as a coordinate transformation of the form

$$x' = Rx \qquad (5.2.1)$$

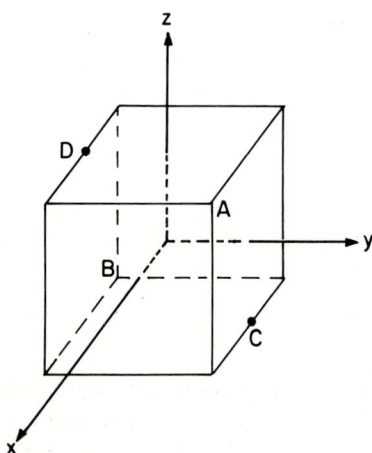

Fig. 5.1. Coordinate system for the cubic group O

in which x and x' are column vectors with components (x, y, z) and (x', y', z') respectively. Associated with R is an operator $P(R)$, defined by the relation

$$P(R)f(x) = f(R^{-1}x). \qquad (5.2.2)$$

Thus, R operates on coordinates while $P(R)$ operates on functions. If the operators R form a group so will the operators $P(R)$, and since the correspondence between the two kinds of operators is one-to-one, the two groups will be isomorphic. This is the basis for the dual interpretations mentioned above.

The characters of the irreducible representations (IR) of the group O are given in Table 5.2. With this table, a reducible representation Γ may be decomposed into irreducible representations $\Gamma^{(i)}$ (for convenience we use superscripts in place of subscripts as in Table 5.2) according to

$$\Gamma = \sum_i a_i \Gamma^{(i)}, \qquad (5.2.3)$$

$$a_i = \frac{1}{h} \sum_R \chi^{(i)}(R)\chi(R). \qquad (5.2.4)$$

Here h is the order of the group; $\chi^{(i)}(R)$ are characters for the operations R in the representation $\Gamma^{(i)}$; $\chi(R)$ are the characters of Γ; and a_i are integers which indicate the number of times a representation $\Gamma^{(i)}$ appears in the decomposition of Γ. The direct product of two IRs is generally reducible; Table 5.3 is a multiplication table which gives the reduction of all possible direct products of two IRs. (The symmetrized products will be described in Section 5.2.3).

Table 5.3. *Multiplication table for the irreducible representations of the cubic group* O

Γ_1	Γ_2	Γ_3	Γ_4	Γ_5	Γ_6	Γ_7	Γ_8	
Γ_1	Γ_2	Γ_3	Γ_4	Γ_5	Γ_6	Γ_7	Γ_8	Γ_1
	Γ_1	Γ_3	Γ_5	Γ_4	Γ_7	Γ_6	Γ_8	Γ_2
		$\Gamma_1+\Gamma_2+\Gamma_3$	$\Gamma_4+\Gamma_5$	$\Gamma_4+\Gamma_5$	Γ_8	Γ_8	$\Gamma_6+\Gamma_7+\Gamma_8$	Γ_3
			$\Gamma_1+\Gamma_3+\Gamma_4+\Gamma_5$	$\Gamma_2+\Gamma_3+\Gamma_4+\Gamma_5$	$\Gamma_6+\Gamma_8$	$\Gamma_7+\Gamma_8$	$\Gamma_6+\Gamma_7+2\Gamma_8$	Γ_4
				$\Gamma_1+\Gamma_3+\Gamma_4+\Gamma_5$	$\Gamma_7+\Gamma_8$	$\Gamma_6+\Gamma_8$	$\Gamma_6+\Gamma_7+2\Gamma_8$	Γ_5
					$\Gamma_1+\Gamma_4$	$\Gamma_2+\Gamma_5$	$\Gamma_3+\Gamma_4+\Gamma_5$	Γ_6
						$\Gamma_1+\Gamma_4$	$\Gamma_3+\Gamma_4+\Gamma_5$	Γ_7
							$\Gamma_1+\Gamma_2+\Gamma_3$ $+2\Gamma_4+2\Gamma_5$	Γ_8

Symmetrized Products:

$[\Gamma_3 \times \Gamma_3] = \Gamma_1 + \Gamma_3$

$[\Gamma_4 \times \Gamma_4] = [\Gamma_5 \times \Gamma_5] = \Gamma_1 + \Gamma_3 + \Gamma_5$

$[\Gamma_6 + \Gamma_6] = [\Gamma_7 \times \Gamma_7] = \Gamma_4$

$[\Gamma_8 \times \Gamma_8] = \Gamma_2 + 2\Gamma_4 + \Gamma_5$

For every irreducible representation, $\Gamma^{(i)}$, in O there are two irreducible representations, $\Gamma_g^{(i)}$ and $\Gamma_u^{(i)}$ in O_h; under inversion the characters of $\Gamma_g^{(i)}$ are positive and those of $\Gamma_u^{(i)}$ negative. $\Gamma_g^{(i)}$ and $\Gamma_u^{(i)}$ are also said to be even and odd representations respectively.

The irreducible representations $D^{(j)}$ of the three-dimensional rotation group R_3 are also representations of O since the latter is a subgroup of R_3; however, with respect to O the $D^{(j)}$ are reducible. The character of a $D^{(j)}$ is given by

$$\chi(\alpha) = \frac{\sin(j+\tfrac{1}{2})\alpha}{\sin\dfrac{\alpha}{2}} \qquad (5.2.5)$$

where α is a rotation about an arbitrary axis. We can then use (5.2.3) and (5.2.4) to establish connections between the irreducible representations in R_3 with those of O; these are shown in Table 5.4. By way of example

$$D^{(2)} = E + T_2 . \qquad (5.2.6)$$

Table 5.4. *Reduction of $D^{(j)}$, the irreducible representations of the three-dimensional rotation group R_3, into the irreducible representations of O*

$D^{(0)}$	A_1	Γ_1
$D^{(1/2)}$	E'	Γ_6
$D^{(1)}$	T_1	Γ_4
$D^{(3/2)}$	U'	Γ_8
$D^{(2)}$	$E + T_2$	$\Gamma_3 + \Gamma_5$
$D^{(5/2)}$	$E'' + U'$	$\Gamma_7 + \Gamma_8$
$D^{(3)}$	$A_2 + T_1 + T_2$	$\Gamma_2 + \Gamma_4 + \Gamma_5$
$D^{(7/2)}$	$E' + E'' + U'$	$\Gamma_6 + \Gamma_7 + \Gamma_8$
$D^{(4)}$	$A_1 + E + T_1 + T_2$	$\Gamma_1 + \Gamma_3 + \Gamma_4 + \Gamma_5$

5.2.2 Basis Functions

The basis functions belonging to a particular representation of a group are defined as a set of functions $\varphi_1^{(k)}, \varphi_2^{(k)} \ldots \varphi_n^{(k)}$ which satisfy linear relations of the form

$$P(R)\varphi_j^{(k)} = \sum_{i=1}^{n} \varphi_i^{(k)} \Gamma_{ij}^{(k)}(R) . \qquad (5.2.7)$$

The $\Gamma_{ij}^{(k)}(R)$ are numerical coefficients; they are components of a matrix $\Gamma^{(k)}(R)$, which is a representation of the group associated with the element R. It is important to note that any member of a basis set when subjected to a symmetry operation according to (5.2.7) yields a linear combination of members of the same set and no other functions. A set of functions which satisfies (5.2.7) is said to transform according to the representation $\Gamma^{(k)}(R)$, or to span or belong to $\Gamma^{(k)}(R)$.

The basis functions for the irreducible representation $D^{(J)}$ of R_3 can be symbolized by $|JM\rangle$ with $J = 0, \tfrac{1}{2}, 1, \tfrac{3}{2}, 2 \ldots$ and $M = J, J-1, \ldots -J$. When J is an integer it is sufficient to regard $|JM\rangle$ as simply the spherical harmonic $Y_{JM}(\theta, \varphi)$, but when J is half integral, $|JM\rangle$ is a spinor. Thus for $J = \tfrac{1}{2}$, the two functions $|\tfrac{1}{2}\tfrac{1}{2}\rangle$ and $|\tfrac{1}{2}-\tfrac{1}{2}\rangle$ are the spin functions α and β. For other half-integral values of J, $|JM\rangle$ can be given an explicit form as a linear combination of products of spherical harmonics and spin functions according to the usual rules for coupling angular momentum eigenfunctions.

Basis functions for the irreducible representations of O can be constructed as linear combinations of $|J M\rangle$. There are many ways of doing this. Thus from Table 5.4, $D^{(2)} = E + T_2$; hence the basis functions for E and T_2 can be constructed as linear combinations of $|2 M\rangle$, i.e. the spherical harmonics Y_{2M}. But higher-order spherical harmonics like $|4 M\rangle$ may serve the same purpose. Similarly, basis functions for U' can be constructed with $|\frac{3}{2} M\rangle$ or $|\frac{5}{2} M\rangle$ as well as higher-order functions. Table 5.5 lists examples of basis functions for the IRs of O which are useful in discussions of d-electron systems. The notation $|\Gamma^{(\alpha)} i\rangle$ identifies the i-th component of a set of basis functions belonging to the irreducible representation $\Gamma^{(\alpha)}$, e.g. $|\Gamma^{(3)} 0\rangle$; in another notation this is $|E \theta\rangle$. Phase conventions and notations are essentially those of GRIFFITH (1961). Of particular interest are the basis sets $(d_{z^2}, d_{x^2-y^2})$ and (d_{xy}, d_{yz}, d_{zx}) which belong to E and T_2 respectively; they are shown in Fig. 5.2. Since O_h contains both even and odd representations, basis functions must also be classified according to their behavior under inversion. Thus $|\Gamma_u^{(\alpha)} i\rangle$ is a basis function which changes sign under

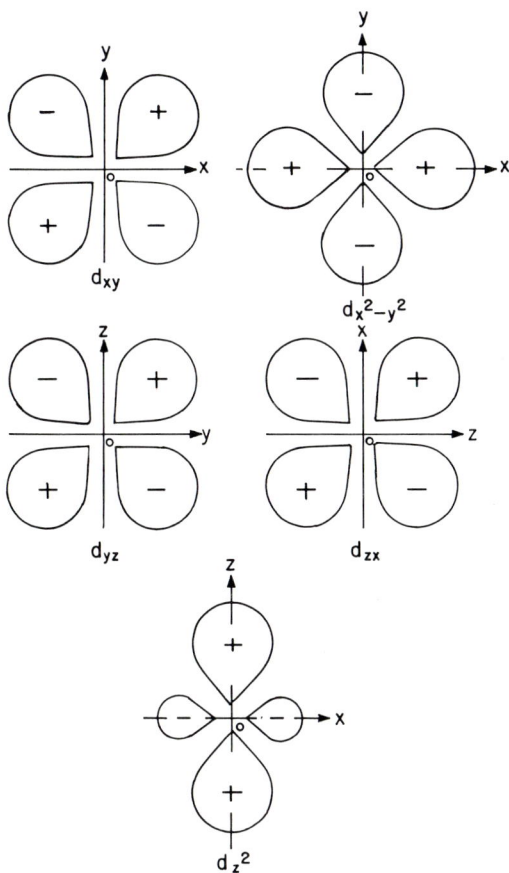

Fig. 5.2. The real d orbitals. $(d_{z^2}, d_{x^2-y^2})$ and (d_{xy}, d_{yz}, d_{zx}) are basis functions for the E and T_2 representations of O respectively

Table 5.5. *Basis functions for the irreducible representations of O*

Irreducible Representations		Basis Functions	

| A_1 | Γ_1 | | $|A_1\rangle = |00\rangle$ | |

| A_2 | Γ_2 | $|A_2\rangle = \dfrac{i}{\sqrt{2}}\,[|3-2\rangle - |32\rangle]$ | $\sqrt{15}\,xyz$ |

| E | Γ_3 | $|E\theta\rangle = |20\rangle$ | $d_{z^2} = \dfrac{1}{2}(3z^2 - r^2) = \sqrt{\dfrac{4\pi}{5}}\,r^3\,|E\theta\rangle$ |
| | | $|E\varepsilon\rangle = \dfrac{1}{\sqrt{2}}\,[|22\rangle + |2-2\rangle]$ | $d_{x^2-y^2} = \dfrac{\sqrt{3}}{2}(x^2 - y^2) = \sqrt{\dfrac{4\pi}{5}}\,r^2\,|E\varepsilon\rangle$ |

For T_1 (Γ_4):

$$|T_1 1\rangle = -\frac{i}{\sqrt{2}}\,[|T_1 x\rangle + i|T_1 y\rangle] \qquad |T_1 x\rangle = \frac{i}{\sqrt{2}}\,[|T_1 1\rangle - |T_1 1\rangle]$$

$$|T_1 0\rangle = i|T_1 z\rangle \qquad |T_1 y\rangle = \frac{1}{\sqrt{2}}\,[|T_1 1\rangle + |T_1 -1\rangle]$$

$$|T_1 -1\rangle = \frac{i}{\sqrt{2}}\,[|T_1 x\rangle - i|T_1 y\rangle] \qquad |T_1 z\rangle = -i|T_1 0\rangle$$

(t_2^4)

$$|{}^3T_1 1x\rangle = |\xi^2 \eta^+ \zeta^+\rangle$$
$$|{}^3T_1 1y\rangle = -|\xi^+ \eta^2 \zeta^+\rangle \qquad [\xi = T_2\xi,\ \eta = T_2\eta,\ \zeta = T_2\zeta]$$
$$|{}^3T_1 1z\rangle = |\xi^+ \eta^+ \zeta^2\rangle$$

For T_2 (Γ_5):

$$|T_2 1\rangle = -\frac{i}{\sqrt{2}}\,[|T_2\xi\rangle + i|T_2\eta\rangle] \qquad |T_2\xi\rangle = \frac{i}{\sqrt{2}}\,[|T_2 1\rangle - |T_2 -1\rangle]$$
$$= |2-1\rangle \qquad\qquad = \frac{i}{\sqrt{2}}\,[|21\rangle + |2-1\rangle]$$

$$|T_2 0\rangle = i|T_2\xi\rangle \qquad |T_2\eta\rangle = \frac{1}{\sqrt{2}}\,[|T_2 1\rangle + |T_2 -1\rangle]$$
$$= \frac{1}{\sqrt{2}}\,[|22\rangle - |2-2\rangle] \qquad\qquad = -\frac{1}{\sqrt{2}}\,[|21\rangle - |2-1\rangle]$$

$$|T_2 -1\rangle = \frac{i}{\sqrt{2}}\,[|T_2\xi\rangle - i|T_2\eta\rangle] \qquad |T_2\zeta\rangle = -i|T_2 0\rangle$$
$$= -|21\rangle \qquad\qquad = -\frac{i}{\sqrt{2}}\,[|22\rangle - |2-2\rangle]$$

$$d_{xy} = \sqrt{3}\,xy = \sqrt{\frac{4\pi}{5}}\,r^2\,|T_2\zeta\rangle$$

$$d_{yz} = \sqrt{3}\,yz = \sqrt{\frac{4\pi}{5}}\,r^2\,|T_2\xi\rangle$$

$$d_{zx} = \sqrt{3}\,zx = \sqrt{\frac{4\pi}{5}}\,r^2\,|T_2\eta\rangle$$

Table 5.5. (continued)

Irreducible Representations	Basis Functions

$$|E'\,\alpha'\rangle = \left|\frac{1}{2}\,\frac{1}{2}\right\rangle$$

E' Γ_6

$$|E'\,\beta'\rangle = \left|\frac{1}{2}-\frac{1}{2}\right\rangle$$

$$|E''\,\alpha''\rangle = \frac{1}{\sqrt 6}\left|\frac{5}{2}\,\frac{5}{2}\right\rangle - \sqrt{\frac{5}{6}}\left|\frac{5}{2}-\frac{3}{2}\right\rangle$$

E'' Γ_7

$$|E''\,\beta''\rangle = \frac{1}{\sqrt 6}\left|\frac{5}{2}-\frac{5}{2}\right\rangle - \sqrt{\frac{5}{6}}\left|\frac{5}{2}\,\frac{3}{2}\right\rangle$$

$$|U'\kappa\rangle = \left|\frac{3}{2}\,\frac{3}{2}\right\rangle \qquad\qquad |U'\kappa\rangle = -\frac{1}{\sqrt 6}\left|\frac{5}{2}\,\frac{3}{2}\right\rangle - \sqrt{\frac{5}{6}}\left|\frac{5}{2}-\frac{5}{2}\right\rangle$$

$$|U'\lambda\rangle = \left|\frac{3}{2}\,\frac{1}{2}\right\rangle \qquad\qquad |U'\lambda\rangle = \left|\frac{5}{2}\,\frac{1}{2}\right\rangle$$

U' Γ_8

$$|U'\mu\rangle = \left|\frac{3}{2}-\frac{1}{2}\right\rangle \qquad\qquad |U'\mu\rangle = -\left|\frac{5}{2}-\frac{1}{2}\right\rangle$$

$$|U'\nu\rangle = \left|\frac{3}{2}-\frac{3}{2}\right\rangle \qquad\qquad |U'\nu\rangle = \sqrt{\frac{5}{6}}\left|\frac{5}{2}\,\frac{5}{2}\right\rangle + \frac{1}{\sqrt 6}\left|\frac{5}{2}-\frac{3}{2}\right\rangle$$

inversion since the notation indicates that it belongs to the odd representation $\Gamma_u^{(\alpha)}$; similarly $|\Gamma_g^\alpha i\rangle$ belongs to the even representation $\Gamma_g^{(\alpha)}$ and does not change sign under inversion.

We shall be dealing with d-electron systems. Since d-orbitals are even under inversion, our main interest is in the even representations of O_h. This is the principal reason why the simpler group O is often used in place of the more cumbersome group O_h.

An illustration of the behavior of basis functions under the operations of the group O may help to clarify the basic ideas. With the z axis along one of the 4-fold symmetry axes as shown in Fig. 5.1, the operation C_4 is taken to be a positive rotation of the coordinate system about the z axis through an angle of $90°$. Then, according to (5.2.1)

$$x' = y, \qquad y' = -x, \qquad z' = z, \tag{5.2.8}$$

and the matrix C_4 connecting x' with x is

$$C_4 = \begin{pmatrix} 0 & 1 & 0 \\ -1 & 0 & 0 \\ 0 & 0 & 1 \end{pmatrix}.$$

From (5.2.2)

$$P(C_4)\,f(x) = f(C_4^{-1}x);$$

this means that $f(x, y, z)$ goes over into $f(-y, x, z)$ under the influence of the coordinate transformation C_4. With the E and T_2 functions given in Table 5.5, we then have

$$
\begin{aligned}
P(C_4)|E\theta\rangle &= |E\theta\rangle, \\
|E\varepsilon\rangle &= -|E\varepsilon\rangle, \\
|T_2\xi\rangle &= |T_2\eta\rangle, \\
|T_2\eta\rangle &= -|T_2\xi\rangle, \\
|T_2\zeta\rangle &= -|T_2\zeta\rangle.
\end{aligned}
\tag{5.2.9}
$$

Alternatively, these relations can be expressed in matrix form,

$$
P(C_4)(E\theta, E\varepsilon) = (E\theta, E\varepsilon)\begin{pmatrix} 1 & 0 \\ 0 & 1 \end{pmatrix},
\tag{5.2.10}
$$

$$
P(C_4)(T_2\xi, T_2\eta, T_2\zeta) = (T_2\xi, T_2\eta, T_2\zeta)\begin{pmatrix} 0 & -1 & 0 \\ 1 & 0 & 0 \\ 0 & 0 & -1 \end{pmatrix}.
\tag{5.2.11}
$$

It is seen, then, that the E functions transform among themselves; hence they satisfy (5.2.7) and in doing so generate a representation of C_4 whose character is zero, as in Table 5.2. Similarly, the T_2 functions transform among themselves and the character of the representation they generate is -1. The same procedure may be repeated with all the elements of the group O to verify that a) the set of E functions do not mix with the set of T_2 functions; each set, when subjected to a symmetry operation mixes only within itself and b) the set of E functions and the set of T_2 functions each generate matrices which are irreducible representations corresponding to E and T_2 respectively, of the group O.

In the discussion of terms in low symmetry fields it is useful to adopt a ket notation of the form $|^{2S+1}hM\theta\rangle$, in which S is the spin quantum number, h is a representation in O, M is the spin-projection quantum number and θ is a component of h. For example $|^2T_2\frac{1}{2}\xi\rangle$ means $S = \frac{1}{2}$, $M = \frac{1}{2}$, the IR of O is T_2 and the component of T_2 is ξ.

5.2.3 Coupling Coefficients

If $D^{(j_1)}$ and $D^{(j_2)}$ are irreducible representations of the three-dimensional rotation group R_3, the product representation, $D^{(j_1)} \times D^{(j_2)}$, is reducible according to

$$
D^{(j_1)} \times D^{(j_2)} = \sum_J D^{(J)}
\tag{5.2.12}
$$

where

$$
J = j_1 + j_2, j_1 + j_2 - 1, \ldots, |j_1 - j_2|.
\tag{5.2.13}
$$

If $|j_1 m_1\rangle$ and $|j_2 m_2\rangle$ are basis sets for $D^{(j_1)}$ and $D^{(j_2)}$ respectively, the basis set, $|JM\rangle$, for any particular $D^{(J)}$ is given by

$$
|JM\rangle = \sum_{m_1, m_2} |j_1 m_1 j_2 m_2\rangle \langle j_1 m_1 j_2 m_2 | JM\rangle.
\tag{5.2.14}
$$

Here

$$M = J, J-1, \ldots, -J = m_1 + m_2,$$

$$|j_1 m_1 j_2 m_2\rangle = |j_1 m_1\rangle |j_2 m_2\rangle.$$

The numerical coefficients $\langle j_1 m_1 j_2 m_2 | J M \rangle$ are known as coupling coefficients; in the specific case of the group R_3, the coefficients are also known as Clebsch-Gordan or Wigner coefficients. (5.2.14) may also be expressed in terms of 3-j symbols which are closely related to the coupling coefficients.

In the same fashion there are coupling coefficients for lower-symmetry groups. Suppose $\Gamma^{(\alpha)}$ and $\Gamma^{(\beta)}$ are irreducible representations of some such group and the corresponding basis sets are $|\Gamma^{(\alpha)} i\rangle$ and $|\Gamma^{(\beta)} j\rangle$. Let $\Gamma^{(\gamma)}$ be one of the IRs contained in the reduction of the product representation $\Gamma^{(\alpha)} \times \Gamma^{(\beta)}$. The basis set $|\Gamma^{(\gamma)} k\rangle$ belonging to the irreducible representation $\Gamma^{(\gamma)}$ then has the form, in analogy with (5.2.14),

$$|\Gamma^{(\gamma)} k\rangle = \sum_{i,j} |\Gamma^{(\alpha)} i \Gamma^{(\beta)} j\rangle \langle \Gamma^{(\alpha)} i \Gamma^{(\beta)} j | \Gamma^{(\gamma)} k\rangle. \tag{5.2.15}$$

The quantities $\langle \Gamma^{(\alpha)} i \Gamma^{(\beta)} j | \Gamma^{(\alpha)} k \rangle$ are the coupling coefficients; tabulations are given by GRIFFITH (1961), KOSTER *et al.* (1963), WATANABE (1966) and others. In using such tabulations it should be kept in mind that the conventions adopted by different authors are not the same. A few examples will help to clarify these matters.

Consider first the $^6A_1$ term. Since $S = \frac{5}{2}$, the spin part of the wave function belongs to $D^{(5/2)}$ of R_3. When the symmetry is reduced to O, the $D^{(5/2)}$ representation decomposes to $E'' + U'$. These may then be coupled with the orbital (space) part of the wave function to produce two product representations: $E'' \times A_1 = E''$ and $U' \times A_1 = U'$. In this case—a rather trivial one—the coupling coefficients are all unity and the basis functions are the ones listed in Table 5.5 for E'' and U' ($J = \frac{5}{2}$). An analogous procedure can be followed for the $^4T_1$ term. Here we have $S = 3/2$ and $D^{(3/2)} = U'$. The product representation, $U' \times T_1 = E' + E'' + 2U'$. When GRIFFITH'S (1961) tables of coupling coefficients are used the basis functions for each of these representations are those shown in Table 5.6. It is interesting to note that in a ^4P state, the spin and orbital parts of the wave function couple with one another to give $J = \frac{1}{2}, \frac{3}{2}, \frac{5}{2}$. In turn $D^{(1/2)} = E'$, $D^{(3/2)} = U'$ and $D^{(5/2)} = E'' + U'$. These are, of course, the same representations as the ones obtained above; it is therefore natural to distinquish the two U' representations by labeling one $J = \frac{3}{2}$ and the other $J = \frac{5}{2}$. These labels appear in Table 5.6.

A single d electron in a cubic field can be found either in an e orbital or in a t_2 orbital. (By analogy with free atoms it is customary to use lower case letters when describing one-electron orbitals; the orbitals ought also to be described more rigorously as e_g and t_{2g}. However, we shall continue to drop the parity index unless it is specifically needed.) If the electron occupies a t_2 orbital, the resulting term is $^2T_2$, where $S = \frac{1}{2}$, $D^{(1/2)} = E'$ and $E' \times T_2 = E'' + U'$. These basis functions, written in several equivalent forms, are also given in Table 5.6. The $\pm$ signs on a one-electron orbital refer to $\alpha(+)$ and $\beta(-)$ spins respectively; $|m^+\rangle = Y_{2m}\alpha$, $|m^-\rangle = Y_{2m}\beta$.

Table 5.6. *Basis functions for the components of the product representations* $U' \times T_1 = E' + E'' + 2U'$ *and* $E' \times T_2 = E'' + U'$. *Coupling coefficients are those of* GRIFFITH *(1961)*

$$|^4T_1 E' \alpha'\rangle = \frac{1}{\sqrt{2}}\left|^4T_1 \frac{3}{2} -1\right\rangle - \frac{1}{\sqrt{3}}\left|^4T_1 \frac{1}{2} 0\right\rangle + \frac{1}{\sqrt{6}}\left|^4T_1 -\frac{1}{2} 1\right\rangle$$

$$|^4T_1 E' \beta'\rangle = \frac{1}{\sqrt{6}}\left|^4T_1 \frac{1}{2} -1\right\rangle - \frac{1}{\sqrt{3}}\left|^4T_1 -\frac{1}{2} 0\right\rangle + \frac{1}{\sqrt{2}}\left|^4T_1 -\frac{3}{2} 1\right\rangle$$

$$|^4T_1 E'' \alpha''\rangle = \frac{1}{\sqrt{6}}\left|^4T_1 \frac{3}{2} 1\right\rangle - \frac{1}{\sqrt{2}}\left|^4T_1 -\frac{1}{2} -1\right\rangle - \frac{1}{\sqrt{3}}\left|^4T_1 -\frac{3}{2} 0\right\rangle$$

$$|^4T_1 E'' \beta''\rangle = -\frac{1}{\sqrt{3}}\left|^4T_1 \frac{3}{2} 0\right\rangle - \frac{1}{\sqrt{2}}\left|^4T_1 \frac{1}{2} 1\right\rangle + \frac{1}{\sqrt{6}}\left|^4T_1 -\frac{3}{2} -1\right\rangle$$

$$|^4T_{1\frac{3}{2}} U' \kappa\rangle = \left(\frac{3}{5}\right)^{\frac{1}{2}}\left|^4T_1 \frac{3}{2} 0\right\rangle - \left(\frac{2}{5}\right)^{\frac{1}{2}}\left|^4T_1 \frac{1}{2} 1\right\rangle$$

$$|^4T_{1\frac{3}{2}} U' \lambda\rangle = \left(\frac{2}{5}\right)^{\frac{1}{2}}\left|^4T_1 \frac{3}{2} -1\right\rangle + \frac{1}{\sqrt{15}}\left|^4T_1 \frac{1}{2} 0\right\rangle - 2\left(\frac{2}{15}\right)^{\frac{1}{2}}\left|^4T_1 -\frac{1}{2} 1\right\rangle$$

$$|^4T_{1\frac{3}{2}} U' \mu\rangle = 2\left(\frac{2}{15}\right)^{\frac{1}{2}}\left|^4T_1 \frac{1}{2} -1\right\rangle - \frac{1}{\sqrt{15}}\left|^4T_1 -\frac{1}{2} 0\right\rangle - \left(\frac{2}{5}\right)^{\frac{1}{2}}\left|^4T_1 -\frac{3}{2} 1\right\rangle$$

$$|^4T_{1\frac{3}{2}} U' \nu\rangle = \left(\frac{2}{5}\right)^{\frac{1}{2}}\left|^4T_1 -\frac{1}{2} -1\right\rangle - \left(\frac{3}{5}\right)^{\frac{1}{2}}\left|^4T_1 -\frac{3}{2} 0\right\rangle$$

$$|^4T_{1\frac{5}{2}} U' \kappa\rangle = -\frac{1}{\sqrt{15}}\left|^4T_1 \frac{3}{2} 0\right\rangle - \frac{1}{\sqrt{10}}\left|^4T_1 \frac{1}{2} 1\right\rangle - \left(\frac{5}{6}\right)^{\frac{1}{2}}\left|^4T_1 -\frac{3}{2} -1\right\rangle$$

$$|^4T_{1\frac{5}{2}} U' \lambda\rangle = \frac{1}{\sqrt{10}}\left|^4T_1 \frac{3}{2} -1\right\rangle + \left(\frac{3}{5}\right)^{\frac{1}{2}}\left|^4T_1 \frac{1}{2} 0\right\rangle + \left(\frac{3}{10}\right)^{\frac{1}{2}}\left|^4T_1 -\frac{1}{2} 1\right\rangle$$

$$|^4T_{1\frac{5}{2}} U' \mu\rangle = -\left(\frac{3}{10}\right)^{\frac{1}{2}}\left|^4T_1 \frac{1}{2} -1\right\rangle - \left(\frac{3}{3}\right)^{\frac{1}{2}}\left|^4T_1 -\frac{1}{2} 0\right\rangle - \left(\frac{1}{10}\right)^{\frac{1}{2}}\left|^4T_1 -\frac{3}{2} 1\right\rangle$$

$$|^4T_{1\frac{5}{2}} U' \nu\rangle = \left(\frac{5}{6}\right)^{\frac{1}{2}}\left|^4T_1 \frac{3}{2} 1\right\rangle + \left(\frac{1}{10}\right)^{\frac{1}{2}}\left|^4T_1 -\frac{1}{2} -1\right\rangle + \left(\frac{1}{15}\right)^{\frac{1}{2}}\left|^4T_1 -\frac{3}{2} 0\right\rangle$$

$$|^2T_2 E'' \alpha''\rangle = \frac{1}{\sqrt{3}}\left|^2T_2 \frac{1}{2} 0\right\rangle - \left(\frac{2}{3}\right)^{\frac{1}{2}}\left|^2T_2 -\frac{1}{2} 1\right\rangle = \frac{1}{\sqrt{3}}|t_2 0^+\rangle - \left(\frac{2}{3}\right)^{\frac{1}{2}}|t_2 1^-\rangle$$

$$= \frac{1}{\sqrt{6}}[|2^+\rangle - |-2^+\rangle] - \left(\frac{2}{3}\right)^{\frac{1}{2}}|-1^-\rangle$$

$$|^2T_2 E'' \beta''\rangle = \left(\frac{2}{3}\right)^{\frac{1}{2}}\left|^2T_2 \frac{1}{2} -1\right\rangle - \frac{1}{\sqrt{3}}\left|^2T_2 -\frac{1}{2} 0\right\rangle = \left(\frac{2}{3}\right)^{\frac{1}{2}}|t_2 -1^+\rangle - \frac{1}{\sqrt{3}}|t_2 0^-\rangle$$

$$= -\left(\frac{2}{3}\right)^{\frac{1}{2}}|1^+\rangle - \frac{1}{\sqrt{6}}[|2^-\rangle - |-2^-\rangle]$$

Table 5.6. (continued)

$$|^2T_2\,U'\kappa\rangle = -\frac{1}{\sqrt{3}}\left|^2T_2\,\tfrac{1}{2}-1\right\rangle-\left(\tfrac{2}{3}\right)^{\frac{1}{2}}\left|^2T_2-\tfrac{1}{2}0\right\rangle = \frac{1}{\sqrt{3}}|t_2-1^+\rangle-\left(\tfrac{2}{3}\right)^{\frac{1}{2}}|t_2 0^-\rangle$$

$$= \frac{1}{\sqrt{3}}|1^+\rangle-\frac{1}{\sqrt{3}}[|2^-\rangle-|-2^-\rangle]$$

$$|^2T_2\,U'\lambda\rangle = \left|^2T_2-\tfrac{1}{2}-1\right\rangle = |t_2-1^-\rangle = -|1^-\rangle$$

$$|^2T_2\,U'\mu\rangle = \left|^2T_2\,\tfrac{1}{2}1\right\rangle = |t_2 1^+\rangle = |-1^+\rangle$$

$$|^2T_2\,U'\nu\rangle = -\left(\tfrac{2}{3}\right)^{\frac{1}{2}}\left|^2T_2\,\tfrac{1}{2}0\right\rangle-\frac{1}{\sqrt{3}}\left|^2T_2-\tfrac{1}{2}1\right\rangle = -\left(\tfrac{2}{3}\right)^{\frac{1}{2}}|t_2 0^+\rangle-\frac{1}{\sqrt{3}}|t_2 1^-\rangle$$

$$= -\frac{1}{\sqrt{3}}[|2^+\rangle-|-2^+\rangle]-\frac{1}{\sqrt{3}}|-1^-\rangle.$$

A common notation for a state in the coupled system is $|^{2S+1}ht\tau\rangle$, in which S is the spin-quantum number, h is a representation in O to which the orbital part of the wave function belongs, t is a representation arising from the coupling of the spin and orbital parts, and τ is a component of t. Thus, $|^4T_1\,E'\alpha'\rangle$ means $S=\tfrac{3}{2}$, the orbital part of the wave function belongs to T_1, E' arises from the coupling of T_1 with $D^{(3/2)}(U')$ and α' is a component of E'.

The case in which the two IRs in a direct product are the same merits additional comment. Suppose, for example, that $(|E\theta_1\rangle,|E\varepsilon_1\rangle)$ and $(|E\theta_2\rangle,|E\varepsilon_2\rangle)$ are two different basis sets each transforming according to the irreducible representation E. The product representation $E\times E$ decomposes (Table 5.3) into A_1+A_2+E, and the basis functions of these IRs can be written with the help of a table of coupling coefficients. They are

$$|A_1\rangle = \frac{1}{\sqrt{2}}[|E\theta_1\rangle|E\theta_2\rangle+|E\varepsilon_1\rangle|E\varepsilon_2\rangle],$$

$$|A_2\rangle = \frac{1}{\sqrt{2}}[|E\theta_1\rangle|E\varepsilon_2\rangle-|E\varepsilon_1\rangle|E\theta_2\rangle|,$$

$$|E\theta\rangle = \frac{1}{\sqrt{2}}[|E\varepsilon_1\rangle|E\varepsilon_2\rangle-|E\theta_1\rangle|E\theta_2\rangle],$$

$$|E\varepsilon\rangle = \frac{1}{\sqrt{2}}[|E\theta_1\rangle|E\varepsilon_2\rangle+|E\varepsilon_1\rangle|E\theta_2\rangle].$$

It is seen that $|A_1\rangle,|E\theta\rangle,|E\varepsilon\rangle$ do not change sign upon interchange of the indices 1 and 2; on the other hand $|A_2\rangle$ does change sign. We therefore refer to A_1 and E as the irreducible representations associated with the decomposition of the *symmetrized* product $[E^2]$. In analogous fashion, A_2 is associated with the *antisymmetrized* product (E^2). When $|E\theta_1\rangle=|E\theta_2\rangle$ and $|E\varepsilon_1\rangle=|E\varepsilon_2\rangle$, i.e. when there is only one basis set, $|A_2\rangle=0$ and we have only components of the symmetrized product. Examples are given in Table 5.3.

5.2.4 Crystal Field Potential

The Hamiltonian of the free ion is spherically symmetric. When the ion is surrounded by a distribution of charges or dipoles, an additional term $V(x)$, which reflects the symmetry of the surrounding distribution, will appear in the Hamiltonian. More precisely, the symmetry group of $V(x)$ is understood to be the group of operators $P(R)$ under whose influence $V(x)$ is an invariant function i. e.

$$P(R)V(x)\equiv V(R^{-1}x)=V(x). \tag{5.2.16}$$

An equivalent statement is that the crystal field potential, $V(x)$, must be a basis function belonging to the totally symmetric representation (A_{1g}) of the symmetry group. The total Hamiltonian is then no longer invariant under all three-dimensional rotations; it is invariant only under the operations of the symmetry group of $V(x)$. We shall now calculate the form of the potential $V_c(x)$ which is invariant under the operations of the cubic group O_h and is appropriate for the description of d-electron systems.

$V_c(x)$ satisfies the Laplace equation, $\nabla^2 V_c(x)=0$, whose general solution for systems in which $r\to0$ is

$$V_c(x)= \sum_{L=0}^{\infty} \sum_{M=-L}^{L} A_{LM}\, r^L\, Y_{LM}(\theta,\varphi). \tag{5.2.17}$$

The origin of the coordinate system (r,ϑ,φ) is taken at the position of the ion nucleus. Since $V_c(x)$ will ultimately be added to the Hamiltonian of the free ion and will be treated as a perturbation, it will be necessary to evaluate matrix elements of $V_c(x)$ taken with respect to the d orbitals of the free ion. According to the Wigner-Eckart theorem

$$\langle Y_{l'm'}|Y_{LM}|Y_{lm}\rangle=(-1)^{m'}\left[\frac{(2l'+1)(2L+1)(2l+1)}{4\pi}\right]^{1/2}$$
$$\times\begin{pmatrix} l' & L & l \\ -m' & M & m \end{pmatrix}\begin{pmatrix} l' & L & l \\ 0 & 0 & 0 \end{pmatrix}. \tag{5.2.18}$$

Therefore, when $l=l'=2$, the first 3-j symbol requires that $(2L2)$ satisfy the triangle relations; this limits the values of L to 0, 1, 2, 3, 4. The second 3-j symbol requires that $2+L+2$ be even; this is equivalent to the requirement that the matrix element be invariant under an inversion in the origin i. e. be of even parity. Hence at this stage the matrix element will vanish unless $L=0, 2$, or 4. The term in (5.2.17) with $L=0$ is a constant; it will have no effect on the free ion states other than to change their energy reference. We therefore eliminate it. The term with $L=2$ is also eliminated because Y_{2M} is not an invariant under O_h. This can be seen from the fact that Y_{2M} belongs to the $D^{(2)}$ representation which reduces in O_h to E_g+T_{2g}. Since the reduction of $D^{(2)}$ into the irreducible representations of O_h does not contain A_{1g}, the totally symmetric representation, there is no combination of basis functions of $D^{(2)}$, i.e. linear combinations of the Y_{2M} which will transform according to A_{1g}. On the other hand, Y_{4M} belongs to $D^{(4)}$, which reduces to $A_{1g} + E_g + T_{1g} + T_{2g}$ (Table 5.4). Since A_{1g} appears in the reduction of $D^{(4)}$, the ligand field potential can be constructed from linear combinations of the Y_{4M}. So far then,

$$V_c(x) = \sum_{M=-4}^{4} A_{4M} r^4 Y_{4M}. \tag{5.2.19}$$

Further restrictions on the form (5.2.19) are obtained by subjecting $V_c(x)$ to various symmetry operations of O and requiring that (5.2.16) be satisfied. The final result, for a real field, is

$$V_c(x) = C r^4 [Y_{40} + \sqrt{\tfrac{5}{14}}(Y_{44} + Y_{4-4})] \tag{5.2.20}$$

or, in Cartesian coordinates,

$$V_c(x) = D(x^4 + y^4 + z^4 - \tfrac{3}{5} r^4) \tag{5.2.21}$$

with

$$D = \frac{15}{4\sqrt{\pi}} C. \tag{5.2.22}$$

The constant D (or C) depends on the disposition of the ligands and their charges (or dipole moments). For point charges of magnitude Ze situated at $(\pm a, 0, 0)$, $(0, \pm a, 0)$ and $(0, 0, \pm a)$ the ligand field potential is

$$V_c(x) = \sum_{\text{ligands}} \frac{Ze^2}{|x - a|}. \tag{5.2.23}$$

When $|x| \ll a$, the binomial expansion of (5.2.23) carried to fourth order gives an expression of the form (5.2.21) with

$$D = \frac{35 Z e^2}{4 a^5}. \tag{5.2.24}$$

From (5.2.22)

$$C = \frac{7\sqrt{\pi} Z e^2}{3 a^5}. \tag{5.2.25}$$

It should be kept in mind that the form of the crystal field potential depends on the choice of axes; the forms given in (5.2.20 or 21) are based on the four-fold axis as the z axis.

5.3 Tetragonal and Rhombic Symmetries

The environment around the iron atom in hemoglobin is never rigorously cubic; in most cases it is necessary to include lower symmetry terms in the Hamiltonian. Next in importance to the cubic term in the crystal field potential is a term having tetragonal (axial) symmetry. For example, the ligands may be located at $x = \pm a$, $y = \pm a$, $z = \pm b$, with $a \neq b$. For such an environment, which departs from cubic symmetry by a distortion along the z axis, it is necessary to include a potential, $V_t(x)$, of the form (Low, 1960; BALLHAUSEN, 1962)

$$V_t(x) = B_2^0(3z^2 - r^2) \tag{5.3.1}$$

in which B_2^0 is a constant, and certain smaller, fourth order terms have been neglected. The potential V_t is invariant under the operations of the group D_4 (or C_{4v}), whose properties are listed in Tables 5.7 and 5.8. There are occasions

Table 5.7. *Symmetry elements and characters of the tetragonal groups D_4 and C_{4v}*

D_4		E	$\bar{E}$	$2C_4$	$2\bar{C}_4$	C_2 $\bar{C}_2$	$2C_2'$ $2\bar{C}_2'$	$2C_2''$ $2\bar{C}_2''$
C_{4v}		E	$\bar{E}$	$2C_4$	$2\bar{C}_4$	C_2 $\bar{C}_2$	$2\sigma_v$ $2\bar{\sigma}_v$	$2\sigma_d$ $2\bar{\sigma}_d$
A_1	Γ_1	1	1	1	1	1	1	1
A_2	Γ_2	1	1	1	1	1	-1	-1
B_1	Γ_3	1	1	-1	-1	1	1	-1
B_2	Γ_4	1	1	-1	-1	1	-1	1
E	Γ_5	2	2	0	0	-2	0	0
E'	Γ_6	1	-2	$\sqrt{2}$	$-\sqrt{2}$	0	0	0
E''	Γ_7	2	-2	$-\sqrt{2}$	$\sqrt{2}$	0	0	0

Definitions (based on the z axis along the 4-fold symmetry axis)

E = identity operation
$\bar{E}$ = rotation through an angle of 2π about an arbitrary axis
C_2 = a rotation of π about the z axis
C_4 = a rotation of $\pm\dfrac{\pi}{2}$ about the z axis
C_2' = a rotation of π about the x or y axis
C_2'' = a rotation of π about an axis inclined at $45°$ to the x and y axis
σ_v = reflection in the xz or yz plane
σ_d = reflection in a plane inclined at $45°$ to both the xz and the yz plane.
A bar over an element indicates multiplication by $\bar{E}$ e. g. $\bar{C}_4 = C_4\bar{E}$.

Table 5.8. *Multiplication table for the irreducible representations of the tetragonal groups D_4 and C_{4v}*

Γ_1	Γ_2	Γ_3	Γ_4	Γ_5	Γ_6	Γ_7	
Γ_2	Γ_3	Γ_4	Γ_5	Γ_6	Γ_7		Γ_1
Γ_1	Γ_4	Γ_3	Γ_5	Γ_6	Γ_7		Γ_2
	Γ_1	Γ_2	Γ_5	Γ_7	Γ_6		Γ_3
		Γ_1	Γ_5	Γ_7	Γ_6		Γ_4
			$\Gamma_1+\Gamma_2+\Gamma_3+\Gamma_4$	$\Gamma_6+\Gamma_7$	$\Gamma_6+\Gamma_7$		Γ_5
				$\Gamma_1+\Gamma_2+\Gamma_5$	$\Gamma_3+\Gamma_4+\Gamma_5$		Γ_6
					$\Gamma_1+\Gamma_2+\Gamma_5$		Γ_7

Symmetrized Products:

$[\Gamma_5 \times \Gamma_5] = \Gamma_1 + \Gamma_3 + \Gamma_4$
$[\Gamma_6 \times \Gamma_6] = [\Gamma_7 \times \Gamma_7] = \Gamma_2 + \Gamma_5$

when terms of still lower symmetry are required; in hemoglobin this is a rhombic term, which, to lowest order, is given by

$$V_r(x) = B_2^2(x^2 - y^2).$$ (5.3.2)

$V_r(x)$ is invariant under the symmetry group D_2 (Tables 5.9 and 5.10).

Table 5.9. *Symmetry elements and characters of the rhombic group D_2*

D_2		E	$\bar{E}$	C_2 $\bar{C}_2$	C_2' $\bar{C}_2'$	C_2'' $\bar{C}_2''$
A_1	Γ_1	1	1	1	1	1
B_2	Γ_2	1	1	-1	1	-1
B_1	Γ_3	1	1	1	-1	-1
B_3	Γ_4	1	1	-1	-1	1
E'	Γ_5	2	-2	0	0	0

E = identity operation
$\bar{E}$ = rotation through an angle of 2π about an arbitrary axis
C_2 = a rotation of π about the z axis
C_2' = a rotation of π about the y axis
C_2'' = a rotation of π about the x axis.

A bar over an element indicates multiplication by $\bar{E}$ e. g., $\bar{C}_2 = C_2\bar{E}$.

Table 5.10. *Multiplication table for irreducible representations of the rhombic group D_2*

Γ_1	Γ_2	Γ_3	Γ_4	Γ_5	
Γ_1	Γ_2	Γ_3	Γ_4	Γ_5	Γ_1
	Γ_1	Γ_4	Γ_3	Γ_5	Γ_2
		Γ_1	Γ_2	Γ_5	Γ_3
			Γ_1	Γ_5	Γ_4
				$\Gamma_1 + \Gamma_2$ $+ \Gamma_3 + \Gamma_4$	Γ_5

An irreducible representation in O is also a representation in D_4 but is generally reducible; similarly an irreducible representation in D_4 is generally reducible in D_2 and so forth. It is therefore possible to trace the genesis of irreducible representations from higher- to lower-symmetry groups. However, some care must be exercised, as can be seen from the group branching diagram.

Thus, D_2 is a subgroup of D_{2h} or D_4; D_4 is a subgroup of D_{4h} or O but C_{4v} is a subgroup of D_{4h} but not of O. Nevertheless, provided we confine ourselves to even representations, the IRs of C_{4v}, D_{4h}, and D_4 are the same. The compatibility relations are shown in Table 5.11.

R_3

O_h

C_{4v} ——————— D_{4h} O

D_{2h} D_4

D_2

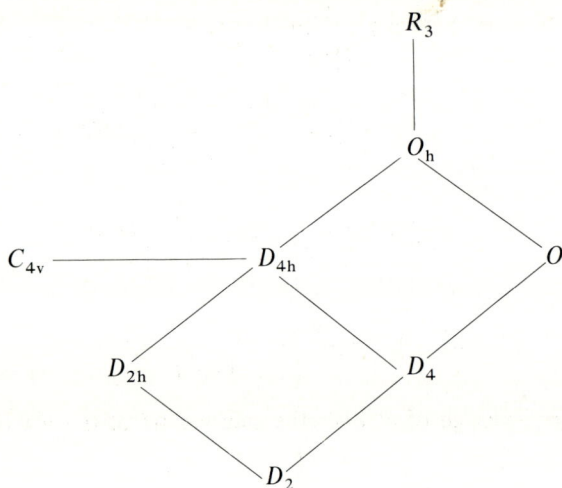

Table 5.11. *Compatibility table for the irreducible representations of O, D_4 (or C_{4v}) and D_2*

O	D_4 or C_{4v}	D_2
A_1	A_1	A_1
A_2	B_1	A_1
E	$A_1(E\,\theta)$	A_1
	$B_1(E\,\varepsilon)$	A_1
T_1	$A_2(T_1 z)$	B_1
	$E(T_1 x, T_1 y$	$B_2 + B_3$
T_2	$B_2(T_2 \zeta)$	B_1
	$E(T_2 \xi, -T_2 \eta)$	$B_2 + B_3$
E'	E'	E'
E''	E''	E'
U'	$E'(U'\lambda, -U'\mu)$	E'
	$E''(-U'\nu, U'\kappa)$	E'

5.4 One-Electron Energies

The five-fold degeneracy of the d orbitals in the free ion, according to (5.2.6), will be partially removed when the ion is placed in a crystal field having cubic symmetry. The same equation tells us that the orbitals will group themselves into a three-fold degenerate set belonging to the t_2 representation and a two-fold degenerate set belonging to the e representation. This is as much information as we can obtain on the basis of group theory alone. To proceed beyond this it is necessary to diagonalize the ligand field potential (5.2.20), using the d orbitals as the basis set. This is readily accomplished with the aid of (5.2.18). Let

$$V_c(m\,m') \equiv \langle \psi_m^d | V_c | \psi_{m'}^d \rangle \qquad (5.4.1)$$

where ψ_m^d represents a d orbital as a product of a radial part and a spherical harmonic Y_{2m} as in (5.1.2). The nonvanishing matrix elements are

$$V_c(00) = \frac{3}{7\sqrt{\pi}} C\langle r^4 \rangle,$$

$$V_c(11) = V_c(-1-1) = -\frac{2}{7\sqrt{\pi}} C\langle r^4 \rangle,$$

$$V_c(22) = V_c(-2-2) = \frac{1}{14\sqrt{\pi}} C\langle r^4 \rangle,$$

$$V_c(2-2) = V_c(-22) = \frac{5}{14\sqrt{\pi}} C\langle r^4 \rangle,$$

where $\langle r^4 \rangle$ is the average of r^4 over the radial part of the wave function. The eigenvalues are

$$E_1 = \frac{3}{7\sqrt{\pi}} C\langle r^4 \rangle,$$

$$E_2 = -\frac{2}{7\sqrt{\pi}} C\langle r^4 \rangle. \qquad (5.4.2)$$

E_1 is 2-fold degenerate and belongs to the e representation, while E_2 is 3-fold degenerate and belongs to the t_2 representations (Fig. 5.3). The difference between

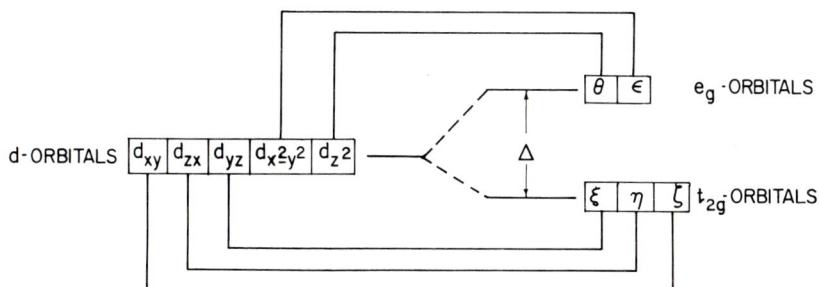

Fig. 5.3. The splitting of d orbitals in an octahedral complex

the two energies, Δ, is the cubic splitting; for 6-fold (octahedral) coordination, (5.2.25) gives

$$\Delta = \frac{5}{3} \frac{Ze^2}{a^5} \langle r^4 \rangle. \qquad (5.4.3)$$

Typical values of Δ for $3d$ electrons are of the order of 10^4 cm^{-1}, with t_2 lower than e when the symmetry is octahedral. These results can also be described in a more pictorial fashion. It is seen from Fig. 5.2 that the $d_{x^2-y^2}$ orbital lies along the x and y axes. This means that an electron in a $d_{x^2-y^2}$ orbital will have a maximum probability density along the coordinate axes, while an electron in a d_{xy} orbital will have maximum probability density along directions which lie at $45°$ to the x and y axes. If the ligands are situated on the axes and are negatively charged, the electrostatic repulsion with an electron in a $d_{x^2-y^2}$ orbital will be greater than with an electron in a d_{xy} orbital. Therefore the energy of the d_{xy} orbital is depressed relative to a $d_{x^2-y^2}$ orbital, as shown in Fig. 5.3. Similar arguments apply to the d_{yz} and d_{zx} orbitals which lie in the yz and zx planes respectively. In addition, since d_{z^2} and $d_{x^2-y^2}$ are degenerate, the same energetic considerations apply to both. We see, then, that states possessing electron distributions which point strongly towards negatively charged regions in the surroundings (e. g. the ligands of a complex) will have a relatively high energy because of the mutual repulsion of negative charges. Others, with electron distributions avoiding the negative charges, will consequently have lower charge.

It is best to keep in mind that a completely literal interpretation of crystal field theory leads to difficulties. The simplicity of Eq. (5.4.3) is deceptive; the cubic splitting can only be obtained from a detailed molecular calculation. Although this has been accomplished in a few instances, more often Δ is treated as an empirical parameter to be obtained from experimental data. In one sense, we can regard crystal field theory as a systematic method for extracting the maximum amount of information from the symmetry properties of the system.

When the symmetry is reduced from cubic to tetragonal there is a further removal of degeneracies. From Table 5.11 we expect the 2-fold degenerate e-orbitals in O to split into two nondegenerate orbitals a_1 and b_1 in D_4. At the

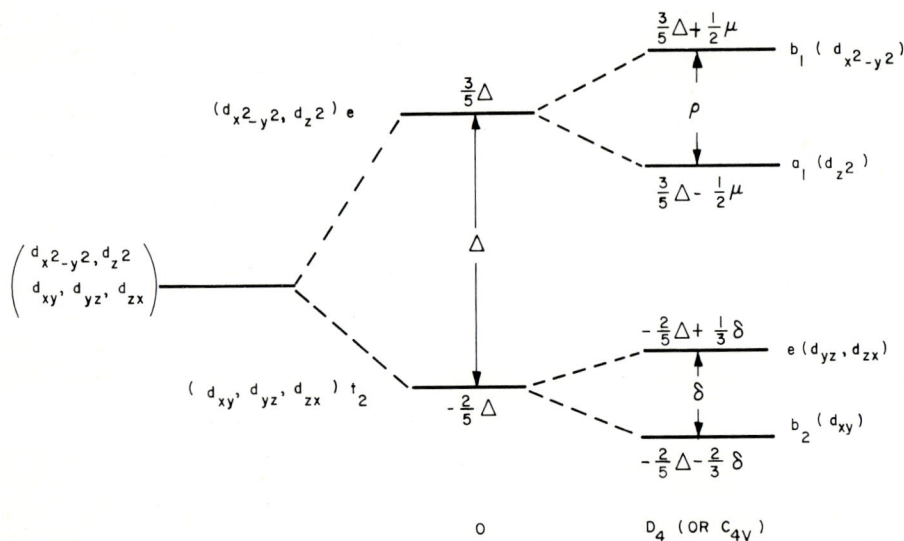

Fig. 5.4. The splitting of d orbitals in a tetragonal field. The negatively charged ligands are at $x = \pm a$, $y = \pm a$, $z = \pm b$ with $b > a$

same time, the 3-fold degenerate t_2-orbitals in O will split into one b_2 (non-degenerate) and one set of e (2-fold degenerate) orbitals; typical energies for the $e-b_2$ separation are of the order of 10^3 cm^{-1}. Fig. 5.4 illustrates these relationships.

In addition to the crystal field potential it is necessary to take into account the effects due to spin-orbit coupling and external magnetic fields. The spin-orbit coupling operator has the form given by (5.1.4). For computational purposes it is generally convenient to adopt a spherical basis in which

$$l_{\pm 1} = \mp \frac{1}{\sqrt{2}}(l_x \pm i l_y), \qquad l_0 = l_z, \tag{5.4.4}$$

$$l_{\pm 1}|l\,m_l\rangle = \mp \left[\frac{l(l+1) - m_l(m_l \pm 1)}{2} \right]^{1/2} |l\,m_l \pm 1\rangle. \tag{5.4.5}$$

Replacing l and m_l by s and m_s gives the corresponding relations for the spin operators. We then have

$$\mathbf{l}\cdot\mathbf{s} = -l_{+1}s_{-1} + l_0 s_0 - l_{-1}s_{+1}. \tag{5.4.6}$$

Table 5.12. *Matrix of* $\mathbf{l}\cdot\mathbf{s}$ *within the set* m^+ *where* $m^+ = Y_{2m}\alpha$ *and* $m^- = Y_{2m}\beta$

$\mathbf{l}\cdot\mathbf{s}$	2^+	1^+	0^+	-1^+	-2^+	2^-	1^-	0^-	-1^-	-2^-
2^+	1									
1^+		$\frac{1}{2}$				1				
0^+			0				$\left(\frac{3}{2}\right)^{\frac12}$			
-1^+				$-\frac{1}{2}$				$\left(\frac{3}{2}\right)^{\frac12}$		
-2^+					-1				1	
2^-		1				-1				
1^-			$\left(\frac{3}{2}\right)^{\frac12}$				$-\frac{1}{2}$			
0^-				$\left(\frac{3}{2}\right)^{\frac12}$				0		
-1^-					1				$\frac{1}{2}$	
-2^-										1

Table 5.13. *Matrix of* $l \cdot s$ *within the set* $\xi^\pm, \eta^\pm, \zeta^\pm$ *where* $(+)$ *and* $(-)$ *refer to* α *and* β *spin respectively*

$l \cdot s$	ξ^+	η^+	ζ^-	ξ^-	η^-	ζ^+
ξ^+		$\dfrac{i}{2}$	$-\dfrac{1}{2}$			
η^+	$-\dfrac{i}{2}$		$\dfrac{i}{2}$			
ζ^-	$-\dfrac{1}{2}$	$-\dfrac{i}{2}$				
ξ^-					$-\dfrac{i}{2}$	$\dfrac{1}{2}$
η^-				$\dfrac{i}{2}$		$\dfrac{i}{2}$
ζ^+				$\dfrac{1}{2}$	$-\dfrac{i}{2}$	

The matrices of $l \cdot s$ in several basis sets are given in Tables 5.12, 5.13 and 5.14. Finally, an external magnetic field whose interaction is described by

$$\mathscr{H}_m = \beta\, H \cdot (l + 2s) \tag{5.4.7}$$

will produce a set of Zeeman levels. These levels are nondegenerate and their characteristics can be investigated by magnetic resonance methods. Matrix elements of $l + 2s$ are given in Tables 5.15 and 5.16. The removal of degeneracies

Table 5.14. *Matrix of* $l \cdot s$ *within the set* $|t_2 1^\pm\rangle, |t_2 0^\pm\rangle, |t_2 -1^\pm\rangle$ *where* $(+)$ *and* $(-)$ *refer to* α *and* β *spin respectively*

$l \cdot s$	$\lvert t_2 1^+\rangle$	$\lvert t_2 0^-\rangle$	$\lvert t_2 -1^+\rangle$	$\lvert t_2 -1^-\rangle$	$\lvert t_2 0^+\rangle$	$\lvert t_2 1^-\rangle$
$\lvert t_2 1^+\rangle$	$-\dfrac{1}{2}$					
$\lvert t_2 0^-\rangle$			$-\dfrac{1}{\sqrt{2}}$			
$\lvert t_2 -1^+\rangle$		$-\dfrac{1}{\sqrt{2}}$	$\dfrac{1}{2}$			
$\lvert t_2 -1^-\rangle$				$-\dfrac{1}{2}$		
$\lvert t_2 0^+\rangle$						$-\dfrac{1}{\sqrt{2}}$
$\lvert t_2 1^-\rangle$					$-\dfrac{1}{\sqrt{2}}$	$\dfrac{1}{2}$

Table 5.15. *Matrices of* $l+2s$ *within the set* $m^{\pm}$ (*notation as in* Table 5.12). *Upper and lower entries refer to x and y components respectively; single entries refer to the z component*

$l+2s$	2^+	1^+	0^+	-1^+	-2^+	2^-	1^-	0^-	-1^-	-2^-
2^+	3	1 $-i$				1 $-i$				
1^+	1 i	2	$\left(\frac{3}{2}\right)^{\frac12}$ $-i\left(\frac{3}{2}\right)^{\frac12}$				1 $-i$			
0^+		$\left(\frac{3}{2}\right)^{\frac12}$ $i\left(\frac{3}{2}\right)^{\frac12}$	1	$\left(\frac{3}{2}\right)^{\frac12}$ $-i\left(\frac{3}{2}\right)^{\frac12}$				1 $-i$		
-1^+			$\left(\frac{3}{2}\right)^{\frac12}$ $i\left(\frac{3}{2}\right)^{\frac12}$	0	1 $-i$				1 $-i$	
-2^+				1 i	-1	0 0				1 $-i$
2^-	1 i				0 0	1	1 $-i$			
1^-		1 i				1 i	0	$\left(\frac{3}{2}\right)^{\frac12}$ $-i\left(\frac{3}{2}\right)^{\frac12}$		
0^-			1 i				$\left(\frac{3}{2}\right)^{\frac12}$ $i\left(\frac{3}{2}\right)^{\frac12}$	-1	$\left(\frac{3}{2}\right)^{\frac12}$ $-i\left(\frac{3}{2}\right)^{\frac12}$	
-1^-				1 i				$\left(\frac{3}{2}\right)^{\frac12}$ $i\left(\frac{3}{2}\right)^{\frac12}$	-2	1 $-i$
-2^-					1 i				1 i	-3

Table 5.16. *Matrices of* $l+2s$ *within the set* $\xi^\pm$, $\eta^\pm$, $\zeta^\pm$ *(notation as in* Table 5.13). *Upper, middle and lower entries are matrix elements of* x, y *and* z *components respectively*

$l+2s$	ξ^+	η^+	ζ^+	ξ^-	η^-	ζ^-
ξ^+				1		
			$-i$	$-i$		
	1	i				
η^+			i		1	
					$-i$	
	$-i$	1				
ζ^+		$-i$				1
	i					$-i$
			1			
ξ^-	1					
	i					$-i$
				-1	i	
η^-		1				i
		i				
				$-i$	-1	
ζ^-			1		$-i$	
			i	i		
						-1

in a $^2T_2$ term by progressive lowering of the symmetry from O to D_4 (or C_{4v}) to D_2 is illustrated in Fig. 5.5; it also shows the effect of spin-orbit and Zeeman interactions on the lowest orbital of $^2T_2$.

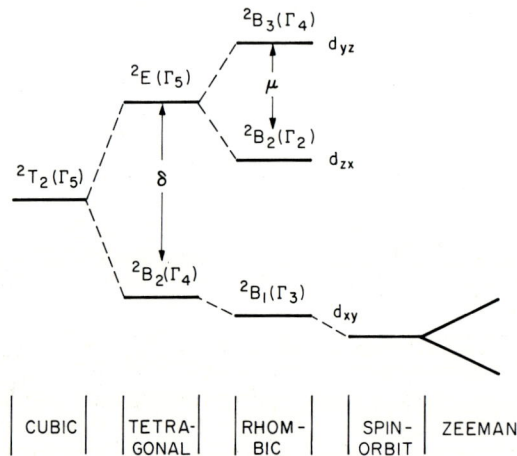

Fig. 5.5. The effect of low symmetry fields, spin-orbit coupling and Zeeman interaction on the $^2T_2$ term

5.5 Multielectron Configurations

An electronic configuration such as $d^5(Fe^{3+})$ or $d^6(Fe^{2+})$ may be subject to the simultaneous presence of Coulombic interactions among the electrons and a crystal field potential (as well as other perturbations which, for the moment, we suppose to be of lesser importance). The relative magnitude of the two inter- actions will determine the sequence in which the Hamiltonian is diagonalized. If the Coulomb interaction predominates, its effect is calculated first; this gives the free ion terms which have already been enumerated for d^5 and d^6 in Table 5.1. The effect of the crystal field such as the cubic field O is then readily determined by consulting Table 5.4. Thus ^6S goes over into $^6A_1$, ^4P into $^4T_1$, ^5D is split into ^5E and $^5T_2$ and so forth. As a check on this procedure the separation between terms should be much larger than any of the splittings due to the crystal field.

If, on the other hand, the crystal field is the dominant interaction the sequence must be reversed. If we confine our attention to a configuration of d electrons and a ligand field of cubic symmetry, the initial effect will be to split the d orbitals into t_2 and e orbitals. For octahedral coordination the t_2 orbitals will lie lower (Section 5.4); their 3-fold degeneracy permits them to be occupied by 6 electrons at most. The e orbitals are 2-fold degenerate; hence they can accommodate a maximum of four electrons. Clearly there are now several possible electronic configurations:

$$d^5(Fe^{3+}): t_2^5, t_2^4 e, t_2^3 e^2, t_2^2 e^3, t_2 e^4,$$

$$d^6(Fe^{2+}): t_2^6, t_2^5 e, t_2^4 e^2, t_2^3 e^3, t_2^2 e^4.$$

These configurations, together with the possible spin alignments corresponding to the maximum value of S, are shown in Fig. 5.6. The configurations listed above

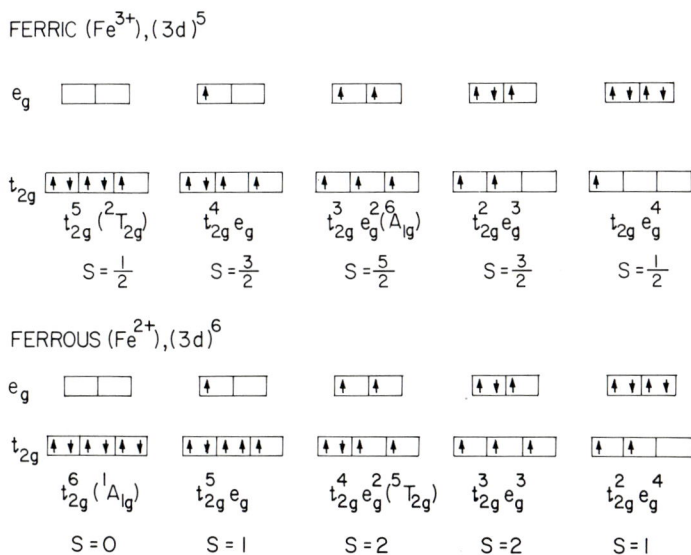

Fig. 5.6. Electronic configurations in t_2 and e orbitals. In each configuration the spin alignment shown is the one that produces the maximum total spin

give rise to a set of terms consistent with the Pauli principle. The situation is precisely analogous to that in the free ion. For example, the configuration t_2^5 leaves a single hole in the t_2 shell; therefore the only possible term from t_2^5 is $^2T_2$. This means that after all five electrons have been coupled to one another the total spin, S, is $1/2$ and the spatial part of the wave function transforms according to the T_2 representation of O. Apart from a few other simple situations it is not possible to obtain the terms arising from a particular configuration merely by inspection. Thus the configuration $t_2^3 e^2$ belongs to the product representation

$$t_2 \times t_2 \times t_2 e \times e,$$

which may be expanded by use of the multiplication table (Table 5.3) into irreducible representations of O. This gives all the possible terms, including some which violate the Pauli principle and must therefore be eliminated. The complete list of strong-field terms (satisfying the Pauli principle) is given in Table 5.17.

The manner in which a configuration like d^5 or d^6 distributes itself among the t_2 and e orbitals is governed by three factors: a) t_2 orbitals lie lower in energy than the e orbitals by an amount Δ; therefore occupation of the t_2 orbitals is favored, b) electrons in the same spatial orbitals tend to have higher electrostatic repulsions than electrons in separate orbitals, and c) exchange energy favors states with high spin, but these, according to the Pauli principle, arise from states in which the electrons are distributed in separate orbitals. The energy associated with the last two factors, taken together, is often called the pairing energy.

Table 5.17. *Terms arising from electronic configurations in a cubic field*

Ferric (Fe^{3+}), $(3d)^5$

Electron Configurations	Terms		
	$S=1/2$	$S=3/2$	$S=5/2$
t_2^5	T_2		
$t_2^4 e$	$A_1\,A_2\,E\,E\,T_1\,T_1\,T_2\,T_2$	$T_1\,T_2$	
$t_2^3 e^2$	$A_1\,A_1\,A_2\,E\,E\,E$ $T_1\,T_1\,T_1\,T_1\,T_2\,T_2\,T_2\,T_2$	$A_1\,A_2\,E\,E\,T_1\,T_2$	A_1
$t_2^2 e^3$	$A_1\,A_2\,E\,E\,T_1\,T_1\,T_2\,T_2$	$T_1\,T_2$	
$t_2 e^4$	T_2		

Ferrous (Fe^{2+}), $(3d)^6$

Electron Configurations	Terms		
	$S=0$	$S=1$	$S=2$
t_2^6	A_1		
$t_2^5 e$	$T_1\,T_2$	$T_1\,T_2$	
$t_2^4 e^2$	$A_1\,A_1\,A_2\,E\,E\,E\,T_1$ $T_2\,T_2\,T_2$	$A_2\,E\,T_1\,T_1\,T_1\,T_2\,T_2$	T_2
$t_2^3 e^3$	$A_1\,A_2\,E\,T_1\,T_1\,T_2\,T_2$	$A_1\,A_2\,E\,E\,T_1\,T_1\,T_2\,T_2$	E
$t_2^2 e^4$	$A_1\,E\,T_2$	T_1	

Hence the relative magnitude of Δ, the orbital separation due to the cubic crystal field, and the pairing energy will determine the distribution of electrons among the t_2 and e orbitals.

Two limiting cases can be distinguished. When Δ is much smaller than the pairing energy, the electrons tend to distribute themselves so as to achieve maximum spin. For Fe^{3+}, the configuration $t_2^3 e^2$ with $S=\frac{5}{2}$ has the lowest energy and for Fe^{2+} it is the configuration $t_2^4 e^2$ with $S=2$ that lies lowest. Conversely, when Δ is much larger than the pairing energy the electrons tend to fill the t_2 orbitals; for Fe^{3+} and Fe^{2+} the lowest energy configurations are $t_2^5(S=\frac{1}{2})$ and $t_2^6(S=0)$ respectively. It is seen, then, that to a large extent, the value of Δ determines the magnetic properties of the complex. In particular, a strong ligand field may produce a diamagnetic ferrous complex, whereas other ferrous complexes possessing weaker ligand fields will consequently be paramagnetic.

As in the case of the free ion, the various terms which result from a particular electronic configuration will differ in energy as a result of Coulombic interactions. These have been calculated by TANABE and SUGANO (1954) as a function of Δ and are expressed in terms of the Racah coefficients. The energies of the lowest states for Fe^{3+} are given by

$$E(t_2^3 e^2, {}^6A_1) = 10A - 35B, \qquad (5.5.1)$$

$$E(t_2^5, {}^2T_2) = 10A - 20B + 10C - 2\Delta, \qquad (5.5.2)$$

$$E(t_2^4 e, {}^4T_1) = 10A - 25B + 6C - \Delta. \qquad (5.5.3)$$

The values of B and C given in Section 5.1 have been used to plot these energies in Fig. 5.7. When $\Delta = 0$, ${}^2T_2$ lies $63\,200$ cm^{-1} above ${}^6A_1$; the two states become equal in energy when

$$\Delta = \Delta_c(Fe^{3+}) = \frac{1}{2}(15B + 10C), \qquad (5.5.4)$$

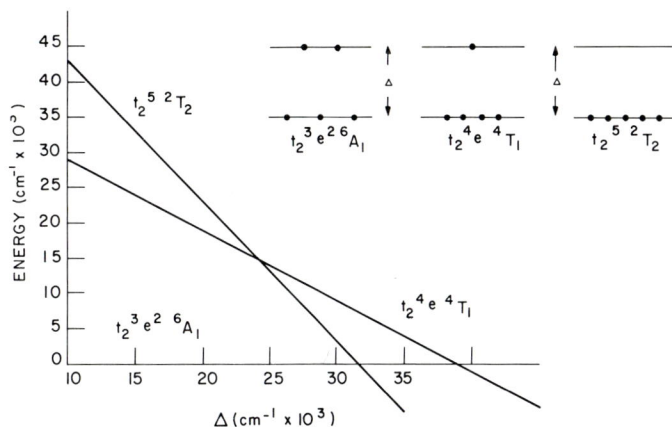

Fig. 5.7. Energies of ${}^2T_2$ and ${}^4T_1$ relative to ${}^6A_1$ for Fe^{3+} as a function of the cubic splitting parameter Δ

which is about $31\,600\;\mathrm{cm}^{-1}$. When values of Δ are greater than Δ_c, $^2T_2$ remains below $^6A_1$. Similarly, $^4T_1$ also crosses $^6A_1$ but never becomes the ground state. For Fe^{2+} the energies of the lowest states are

$$E(t_2^6, {}^1A_1) = 15\,A - 30\,B + 15\,C, \tag{5.5.5}$$

$$E(t_2^4 e^2, {}^5T_2) = 15\,A - 35\,B + 7\,C + 2\Delta, \tag{5.5.6}$$

and the energy separation between $^1A_1$ and $^5T_2$, when $\Delta = 0$, is $37000\;\mathrm{cm}^{-1}$; the cross-over occurs when

$$\Delta = \Delta_c(Fe^{2+}) = \tfrac{1}{2}(5\,B + 8\,C), \tag{5.5.7}$$

which is about $18\,500\;\mathrm{cm}^{-1}$ (Fig. 5.8).

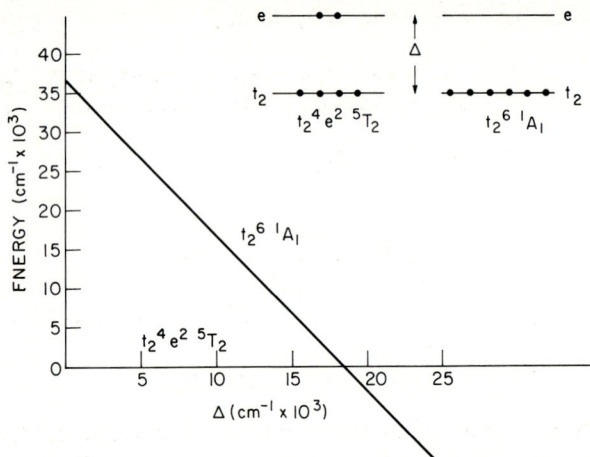

Fig. 5.8. Energy of $^1A_1$ relative to $^5T_2$ for Fe^{2+} as a function of the cubic splitting parameter Δ

It is often desirable to express a term as an expansion of one-electron orbitals. For example, the $^2T_2$ term of t_2^5 has one unoccupied t_2 orbital; therefore

$$|t_2^5\,{}^2T_2\tfrac{1}{2}\zeta\rangle = |\xi^+\,\eta^2\,\zeta^2\rangle,$$
$$|t_2^5\,{}^2T_2\tfrac{1}{2}\eta\rangle = |\xi^2\,\eta^+\,\zeta^2\rangle, \tag{5.5.8}$$
$$|t_2^5\,{}^2T_2\tfrac{1}{2}\zeta\rangle = |\xi^2\,\eta^2\,\zeta^+\rangle.$$

The kets on the right may be interpreted as 5×5 Slater determinants when it is necessary to satisfy antisymmetry requirements. For $^4T_1$ from $t_2^4 e$ the situation is a little more complicated. A single electron in an e orbital can produce only one term, ^2E, so that

$$|e^2 E \tfrac{1}{2}\theta\rangle = |\theta^+\rangle,$$
$$|e^2 E \tfrac{1}{2}\varepsilon\rangle = |\varepsilon^+\rangle. \tag{5.5.9}$$

The four electrons which make up t_2^4 produce $^1A_1$, ^1E, $^1T_2$ and $^3T_1$ (GRIFFITH, 1961). These states coupled with ^2E must produce $^4T_1$; clearly it is only the triplet state $^3T_1$ which can combine with the doublet ^2E to form the quartet $^4T_1$. This is expressed by writing the term as $|t_2^4(^3T_1)e(^2E)^4T_1\rangle$. From Table 5.5

$$|t_2^4\,{}^3T_1\,1\,x\rangle=|\xi^2\,\eta^+\,\zeta^+\rangle,$$

$$|t_2^4\,{}^3T_1\,1\,y\rangle=-|\xi^+\,\eta^2\,\zeta^+\rangle, \qquad (5.5.10)$$

$$|t_2^4\,{}^3T_1\,1\,z\rangle=|\xi^+\,\eta^+\,\zeta^2\rangle.$$

When (5.5.9) and (5.5.10) are combined by means of the coupling coefficients, we have

$$|t_2^4(^3T_1)e(^2E)^4T_1\tfrac{3}{2}x\rangle=-\tfrac{1}{2}|\xi^2\eta^+\zeta^+\theta^+\rangle+\tfrac{1}{2}\sqrt{3}|\xi^2\eta^+\zeta^+\varepsilon^+\rangle,$$

$$|t_2^4(^3T_1)e(^2E)^4T_1\tfrac{3}{2}y\rangle=\tfrac{1}{2}|\xi^+\eta^2\zeta^+\theta^+\rangle+\tfrac{1}{2}\sqrt{3}|\xi^+\eta^2\zeta^+\varepsilon^+\rangle, \qquad (5.5.11)$$

$$|t_2^4(^3T_1)e(^2E)^4\,T_1\tfrac{3}{2}z\rangle=|\xi^+\eta^+\zeta^2\theta^+\rangle.$$

Finally, for $^6A_1$ from $t_2^3e^2$, all five electrons must have parallel spin; hence can be only one electron in each of the five orbitals. This leads to

$$|t_2^3(^4A_2)e^2(^3A_2)^6A_1\tfrac{5}{2}\rangle=-|\xi^+\,\eta^+\,\zeta^+\,\theta^+\,\varepsilon^+\rangle. \qquad (5.5.12)$$

5.6 Kramers Theorem

We define an operator K, sometimes called the time-reversal or the Kramers operator, by

$$K f(x,\,t)=f^*(x,\,-t)$$

i.e. the effect of K on a function of position coordinates, x, and the time, t, is to reverse the sign of t and to take the complex conjugate. If $\mathcal{H}(x)$ is a Hamiltonian operator which is a real function of x and independent of the time, then $K\mathcal{H}(x)\psi(x,t)$ $=\mathcal{H}^*(x)\psi^*(x,\,-t)=\mathcal{H}(x)K\psi(x,t)$. Since $K\mathcal{H}\psi=K\mathcal{H}K^{-1}K\psi$, we have $K\mathcal{H}K^{-1}=\mathcal{H}$ or

$$K\mathcal{H}=\mathcal{H}K. \qquad (5.6.1)$$

If $\psi(x,t)$ satisfies the Schrodinger equation

$$\mathcal{H}(x)\psi(x,\,t)=i\hbar\,\frac{\partial}{\partial t}\,\psi(x,\,t), \qquad (5.6.2)$$

then (5.6.1) implies that $K\psi$ is also a solution, i.e.

$$\mathcal{H}(x)K\psi(x,\,t)=i\hbar\,\frac{\partial}{\partial t}\,K\psi(x,\,t). \qquad (5.6.3)$$

The angular momentum operator, L, is imaginary; hence

$$KL=-LK \qquad (5.6.4)$$

but, because of (5.6.1), $KL\cdot S=L\cdot SK$. Therefore

$$KS=-SK. \qquad (5.6.5)$$

It is now possible to establish the effect of K on the spin functions α and β. Since $S_z \alpha = \frac{1}{2}\alpha$ and $K S_z \alpha = \frac{1}{2} K \alpha$, then, because of (5.6.5)

$$S_z(K\alpha) = -\frac{1}{2}(K\alpha). \qquad (5.6.6)$$

Similarly

$$S_z(K\beta) = \frac{1}{2}(K\beta). \qquad (5.6.7)$$

We see, then, that $K\alpha$ behaves like β and $K\beta$ like α. Eqs. (5.6.6) and 5.6.7) can be satisfied by choosing

$$K\alpha = i\beta,$$

$$K\beta = -i\alpha.$$

or, combining the two relations,

$$K|m_s\rangle = (-1)^{m_s}|-m_s\rangle. \qquad (5.6.8)$$

Suppose now we have a one-electron wave function $\psi = |n l m_l m_s\rangle$ which satisfies the Schrodinger equation and whose spatial part has the form (5.1.2). Then

$$K\psi = K|n l m_l m_s\rangle = (-1)^{m_l + m_s}|n l -m_l -m_s\rangle. \qquad (5.6.9)$$

The two solutions ψ and $K\psi$ must be independent, as otherwise it would be possible to write $K\psi = a\psi$ where a is a constant, or $K^2\psi = a^* a\psi$. But, from (5.6.9), $K^2\psi = -\psi$. Since $a^* a$ cannot be -1, ψ and $K\psi$ must be independent solutions and the state in question is 2-fold degenerate. The same argument can be extended to any odd number of electrons; however, it is not valid for an even number of electrons. Thus, suppose we have a two-electron wave function, say $\psi_1 \psi_2$. This time, it follows from (5.6.9) that $K^2 \psi_1 \psi_2 = \psi_1 \psi_2$, so that it is possible to satisfy $K\psi_1 \psi_2 = a\psi_1 \psi_2$ because $K^2 \psi_1 \psi_2 = a^* a \psi_1 \psi_2$ and $a^* a = 1$. This means that $K\psi_1 \psi_2$ and $\psi_1 \psi_2$ need not be independent. The results we have just obtained are not valid when a magnetic field is present. This can be seen from the form of the Hamiltonian (5.4.7), which does not commute with the operator K. Therefore it is no longer necessary for $K\psi$ to be a solution of the Schrodinger equation when ψ is a solution.

The general conclusions are that in the absence of a magnetic field, the states of a system containing an odd number of electrons will have at least 2-fold degeneracies, no matter how low the symmetry of the crystal field. For a system containing an even number of electrons, the theorem does not apply and a crystal field can remove degeneracies completely. When a magnetic field is present, degeneracies can be completely removed in systems containing either an odd or an even number of electrons.

From (5.6.9) and Table 5.5 it is easily verified that

$$K|\xi^+\rangle = i|\xi^-\rangle, \quad K|\xi^-\rangle = -i|\xi^+\rangle,$$

$$K|\eta^+\rangle = i|\eta^-\rangle, \quad K|\eta^-\rangle = -i|\eta^+\rangle, \qquad (5.6.10)$$

$$K|\zeta^+\rangle = i|\zeta^-\rangle, \quad K|\zeta^-\rangle = -i|\zeta^+\rangle.$$

5.7 The Jahn-Teller Effect

According to the Jahn-Teller theorem (see also Section 9.2) a symmetric (nonlinear) molecule in a degenerate electronic state (other than Kramers degeneracy) is unstable aginst distortions of the nuclear framework which reduce the symmetry and remove the degeneracy (STURGE, 1967; ABRAGAM and BLEANEY, 1970; HAM, 1972; ENGLMAN, 1972). In other words, there is a state of lower energy for a less symmetrical configuration. The theorem also prescribes the kinds of distortions that occur: if the electronic state of the symmetric molecule belongs to the irreducible representation Γ, then the symmetry species of the possible Jahn-Teller distortions are the components of the symmetrized product $[\Gamma^2]$, except for the totally symmetric representation (A_{1g}).

Suppose, for example, that the electronic state of the molecule is E_g (octahedral symmetry, group O_h), then since $[E_g^2] = A_{1g} + E_g$, as indicated in Table 5.3, the symmetry species of the distortion will be ε_g. (We use Greek letters to describe nuclear symmetries to avoid confusion with electronic symmetries). In Section 9.2 this type of distortion is examined in greater detail and is shown to correspond to a reduction in symmetry from O_h to D_{4h}. In a similar fashion, if the electronic symmetry is T_{2g}, since $[T_{2g}^2] = A_{1g} + E_g + T_{2g}$, the Jahn-Teller distortions or deformations modes belong to ε_g or τ_{2g}. The latter corresponds to a trigonal (D_{3d}) distortion.

The magnitude of the effect depends on the strength of the coupling between electronic and nuclear motions. If the coupling is sufficiently strong the molecule will undergo a static distortion; if, however, the coupling is so weak that the gain in energy from the Jahn-Teller distortion is of the same order of magnitude as the zero-point energy of the associated vibrational mode, dynamic effects may occur but static distortions will not be observed except perhaps at very low temperatures.

5.8 Molecular Orbitals

We have noted that crystal field theory deals entirely with the properties of the orbitals associated with the central ion. The effect of the ligands is reflected in a crystal field potential which is added to the Hamiltonian of the free ion. In the molecular orbital approach the ligands and the central ion are treated on an equal footing. Linear combinations of ligand orbitals with central ion orbitals are constructed to produce a set of molecular orbitals which may be bonding, nonbonding, or antibonding. The characterization of a complex as "ionic" or "covalent" now becomes a matter of the relative magnitude of the coefficients of cation vs ligand orbitals. Since both the ligands and the central ion contribute electrons to populate the molecular orbitals such electrons can generally no longer be considered as localized either on the ligands or on the central ion. Rather, the coefficients in the molecular orbitals determine the probability of finding an electron in a particular location. One then attempts to understand the physical properties of the complex in terms of the molecular orbitals and the distribution of electrons within them.

The molecular orbital method applied to complexes may be illustrated by reference to a complex of the form MX_6 with symmetry O_h (BALLHAUSEN, 1962; SCHOFFA, 1964; BALLHAUSEN and GRAY, 1965; WATANABE, 1966). The six ligands $X_1...X_6$ can form both σ and π coordinations with the central ion M, which we take to be Fe. The previous discussions dealt entirely with the $3d$ orbitals; for molecular orbital calculations we must augment these with $4s$ and $4p$ orbitals, which can also form σ and π bonds with ligand orbitals. The classification according to O_h is given by

$$a_{1g}: 4s,$$
$$t_{1u}: 4p_x, 4p_y, 4p_z,$$
$$e_g: d_{z^2}, d_{x^2-y^2},$$
$$t_{2g}: d_{xy}, d_{yz}, d_{zx}.$$

The ligand s and p orbitals are similarly organized into linear combinations which transform according to representations of O_h; such linear combinations are often called symmetry orbitals. Metal-ion orbitals and ligand-symmetry orbitals which have the same transformation properties are finally combined linearly to form molecular orbitals.

Ligand orbitals of the σ type are wave functions whose maxima are oriented in the direction of the central ion (Fig. 5.9). Such orbitals may be arranged into linear combinations which transform according to the irreducible representations a_{1g}, e_g and t_{1u} of O_h, as shown in Table 5.18. These will then be the ligand symmetry orbitals which will form σ bonds with orbitals of the central ion which

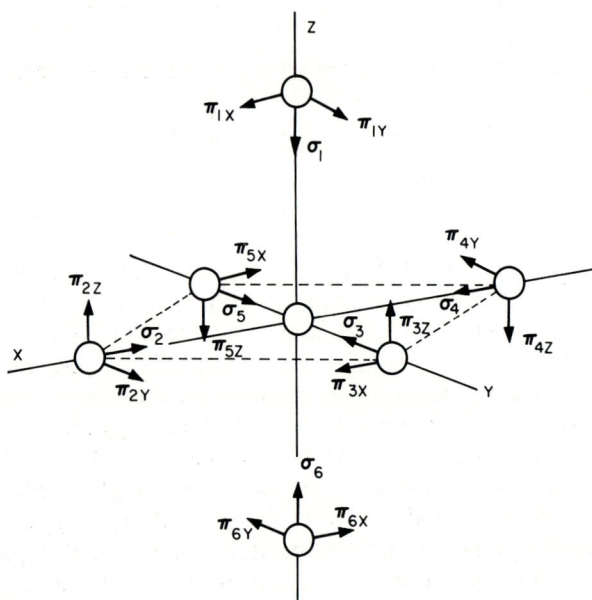

Fig. 5.9. Coordinate system for σ and π orbitals in an octahedral complex

Table 5.18. *Ligand symmetry orbitals for an octahedral complex, group O_h*

		σ	π
a_{1g}	$4s$	$\frac{1}{\sqrt{6}}(\sigma_1+\sigma_2+\sigma_3+\sigma_4+\sigma_5+\sigma_6)$	
e_g	$3d_{z^2}$	$\frac{1}{\sqrt{12}}(2\sigma_1+2\sigma_6-\sigma_2-\sigma_3-\sigma_4-\sigma_5)$	
	$3d_{x^2-y^2}$	$\frac{1}{2}(\sigma_2+\sigma_4-\sigma_3-\sigma_5)$	
t_{1u}	$4p_x$	$\frac{1}{\sqrt{2}}(\sigma_2-\sigma_4)$	$\frac{1}{2}(\pi_{3x}-\pi_{5x}+\pi_{1x}-\pi_{6x})$
	$4p_y$	$\frac{1}{\sqrt{2}}(\sigma_3-\sigma_5)$	$\frac{1}{2}(\pi_{2y}-\pi_{4y}+\pi_{1y}-\pi_{6y})$
	$4p_z$	$\frac{1}{\sqrt{2}}(\sigma_1-\sigma_6)$	$\frac{1}{2}(\pi_{2z}-\pi_{4z}+\pi_{3z}-\pi_{5z})$
t_{2g}	$3d_{xy}$		$\frac{1}{2}(\pi_{2y}+\pi_{3x}+\pi_{4y}+\pi_{5x})$
	$3d_{yz}$		$\frac{1}{2}(\pi_{2x}+\pi_{4x}+\pi_{1x}+\pi_{6x})$
	$3d_{xz}$		$\frac{1}{2}(\pi_{3z}+\pi_{5z}+\pi_{1y}+\pi_{6y})$

belong to the same irreducible representation. An example of a σ type molecular orbital would be

$$\psi_{x^2-y^2}=\alpha d_{z^2}+\beta\left[\tfrac{1}{2}(\sigma_2+\sigma_4-\sigma_3-\sigma_5)\right]$$

where α and β are mixing coefficients.

The case in which $\alpha=1$ and $\beta=0$ represents that of the pure crystal field or the purely ionic bond; as α gets smaller (and β larger) the covalency is increased.

Ligand orbitals of the π type are oriented at right angles to the σ orbitals (Fig. 5.9) and the possible symmetries for this case are t_{1g}, t_{1u}, t_{2g} and t_{2u}, as shown in more detail in Table 5.18. As before, molecular orbitals are constructed as linear combinations of a ligand-symmetry orbital (π type) and a central-ion orbital, both of them belonging to the same irreducible representation. This results in the formation of a π bond. A schematic energy level diagram for both σ and π bonds in an octahedral complex is shown in Fig. 5.10. We note the presence of σ bonding $[a_{1g}(\sigma), e_g(\sigma), t_{1u}(\sigma)]$, σ-antibonding $[a_{1g}(\sigma^*), e_g(\sigma^*), t_{1u}(\sigma^*)]$, π-bonding $[t_{2g}(\pi), t_{1u}(\pi)]$ and π-antibonding $[t_{2g}(\pi^*), t_{1u}(\pi^*)]$ orbitals. In addition, there are two ligand-symmetry orbitals—$t_{1g}(\pi^0)$ and $t_{2u}(\pi^0)$—which do not participate in the formation of molecular orbitals because the central ion has no orbitals belonging to t_{1g} or t_{2u}. It is therefore appropriate to describe $t_{1g}(\pi^0)$ and $t_{2u}(\pi^0)$ as nonbonding, with the consequence that electrons in these orbitals

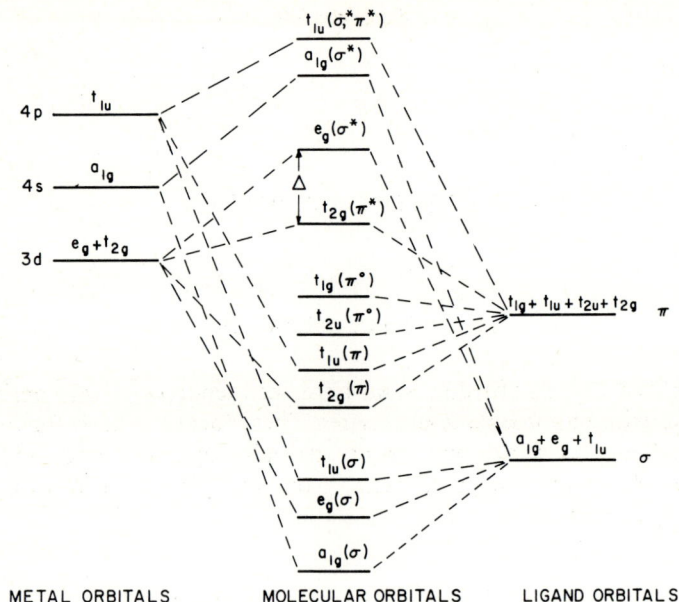

Fig. 5.10. Molecular orbitals for an octahedral complex

are confined to the vicinity of the ligands. Typically, the mixing coefficients are such that the bonding orbitals are mainly those belonging to the ligands while $t_{2g}(\pi^*)$ and $e_g(\sigma^*)$ are mainly those of the ion.

Previously it was pointed out that the electrostatic repulsion between electrons in an orbital like $d_{x^2-y^2}$ (or d_{z^2}) and the negatively charged ligands raises the energy of such orbitals relative to the set d_{xy}, d_{yz} and d_{zx}. On the basis of the molecular orbital approach the increase in energy is associated with the formation of an antibonding $e_g(\sigma^*)$ orbital which is raised in energy by an amount Δ relative to the weekly antibonding $t_{2g}(\pi^*)$ orbital.

Electrons originally belonging to the ion as well as those belonging to the ligands are placed into the lowest orbitals until all the electrons have been accommodated. Each ligand usually supplies two σ electrons and four π electrons, making a total of 36 electrons which completely fill the bonding and nonbonding orbitals $[a_{1g}(\sigma), e_g(\sigma), t_{1u}(\sigma), t_{2g}(\pi), t_{1u}(\pi), t_{2u}(\pi^0)$ and $t_{1g}(\pi^0)]$. Electrons from the ion are accommodated in $t_{2g}(\pi^*)$ and $e_g(\sigma^*)$.

Chapter VI

Magnetic Properties

6.1 General Features

The unfilled d shell of iron, as we have seen, endows certain derivatives of hemoglobin with paramagnetic properties. These form the basis for two experimental methods—electron-spin resonance and magnetic susceptibility—from which most of our knowledge concerning the low-lying states of iron in hemoglobin has been derived.

6.1.1 Electron Spin Resonance

In a typical electron-spin resonance (ESR)—also known as electron paramagnetic resonance (EPR)—experiment, the sample under study is exposed simultaneously to a constant magnetic field and electromagnetic waves at a fixed frequency in the microwave region (e.g. X band). The magnetic field is slowly varied in search of resonances which are first derivatives of characteristic absorptions of microwave energy; a plot of the derivative signals as a function of magnetic field constitutes the most common type of ESR spectrum. When the resonances are well-resolved, their positions on the magnetic field axis are described by g values defined by

$$g = \frac{\hbar \omega}{\beta H} = 0.712 \times 10^{-6} \frac{v}{H} \qquad (6.1.1)$$

(see, for example, ABRAGAM and BLEANEY, 1970), where $\hbar \omega$ is the energy of a microwave photon, $v = \omega/2\pi$ is the microwave frequency (Hz), H is the magnetic field (gauss) and β is the Bohr magneton:

$$\beta = \frac{e\hbar}{2mc} = 0.9271 \times 10^{-20} \text{ erg/gauss} .$$

For a free electron, $g = g_e = 2.0023$; this is the free-spin value for which (6.1.1) becomes

$$\text{(free spin)} \quad \frac{v}{H} = 2.81 \text{ MHz/gauss} . \qquad (6.1.2)$$

It is quite common for the g value to deviate from the free spin-value and in the most general case g is a symmetric tensor of rank two. In an appropriate coordinate system there are three principal values, which can differ from one another, depending on the direction of the magnetic field. We note that the description of a spin resonance experiment by means of a g value implies a direct proportionality between microwave frequency and magnetic field.

An important advantage of the ESR method is that it is applicable to samples in various forms, e.g. single crystal, powder, solution. In hemoglobin the spin-lattice relaxation time is sufficiently short at room temperature to cause serious line broadening; it is therefore necessary to perform ESR measurements at cryogenic temperatures. Examples of ESR spectra in hemoglobin are shown in Figs. 6.1 and 6.2.

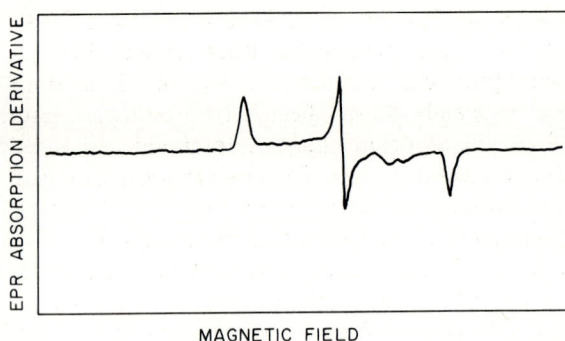

Fig. 6.1. ESR spectrum of a low-spin ($S=\frac{1}{2}$) hemoglobin derivative (BLUMBERG and PEISACH, 1971)

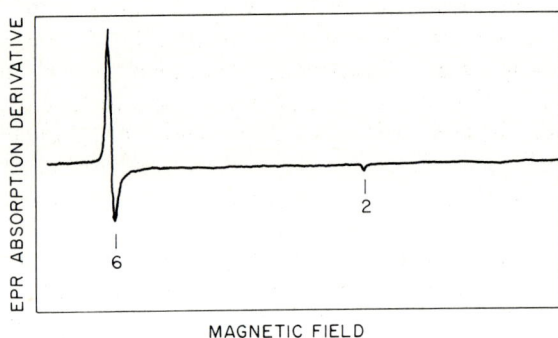

Fig. 6.2. ESR spectrum of a high-spin ($S=\frac{5}{2}$) hemoglobin derivative (PEISACH et al., 1971)

The paramagnetic properties of hemoglobin have their origin in the various possible spin alignments of the $3d$ electrons in iron as shown in Fig. 5.6, but as we have previously noted (Section 2.2), ferric derivatives of hemoglobin have $S=\frac{1}{2}$ or $\frac{5}{2}$ (but not $\frac{3}{2}$) and ferrous derivatives have $S=0$ or 2 (but not 1). Arguments for the absence of compounds with intermediate values of spin have been developed on energetic grounds (GRIFFITH, 1956a; ZERNER et al., 1966; see also Section 7.2). The ferric derivatives are therefore paramagnetic, and ESR spectra have been observed in such compounds. Among ferrous hemoglobins, the low-spin ($S=0$) variety is diamagnetic; hence we do not expect to see any ESR signals but neither have they been observed in high-spin ($S=2$) deoxyhemoglobin.

A possible reason for this is that Kramers' theorem does not apply to systems with an even number of electrons, such as the $(3d)^6$ configuration in ferrohemoglobin. A sufficiently asymmetric crystal field may therefore remove all degeneracies so that none are left to be removed by a magnetic field. In such a system, electron-spin resonance is not likely to be observed except when two levels fortuitously come sufficiently close to one another for a microwave photon to induce a transition. Alternatively or additionally, it is quite possible that the absence of ESR signals in deoxyhemoglobin is attributable to a very short spin-lattice relaxation time.

The interpretations of ESR experiments in hemoglobin have been based on crystal field theory, for which some of the formalism has already been developed in Chapter 5. In this approach, attention is focused on the central ion surrounded by a configuration of ligands whose effect is to produce a perturbing potential at the position of the ion. Symmetry plays a dominant role and the altered properties of the complex relative to the free ion are seen as consequences of the changes in energy and occupation of the orbitals as brought about by the influence of the crystal field. In its simplest form, crystal field theory ignores the possibility of electronic charge being exchanged between the central ion and the ligands; in other words, the $3d$ electrons in iron are presumed to be localized on their parent iron atom. Molecular orbital calculations (see Chapter 7) indicate that this is only approximately true; nevertheless, as we shall see, the assumption of localized atomic orbitals suffices for the description of magnetic properties. It should be mentioned, however, that for other properties, such as optical spectra and Mossbauer resonance, it is necessary to employ the more detailed molecular orbital calculations or to introduce additional parameters into the crystal field theory in order to account for delocalization. The dominant symmetry around the iron atom in hemoglobin is cubic (octahedral); hence it is appropriate to label the electronic states according to the irreducible representations of the cubic group O. However a satisfactory interpretation of experimental data requires that lower symmetry terms be included in the crystal field potential.

The first few electronic states of iron in hemoglobin are shown in Fig. 5.7 for ferric derivatives and in Fig. 5.8 for ferrous. There is a good deal of similarity between the two types. In each case the ground state has a high spin when Δ, the cubic splitting parameter, is small; the nearest excited low-spin state is then relatively far removed. Thus, when $\Delta = 0$, the ferric ground state is $^6A_1$ and the low-spin state, $^2T_2$, lies $63\,200\ \text{cm}^{-1}$ higher; the ferrous ground state is $^5T_2$ and $37\,000\ \text{cm}^{-1}$ above it is $^1A_1$. As Δ increases, the high- and low-spin states approach one another and eventually cross, so that beyond a critical value, $\Delta = \Delta_c$, the ground state takes on a low spin. Hemoglobin derivatives, both ferric and ferrous, appear to be characterized by a value of Δ approximately equal to Δ_c, that is, high- and low-spin derivatives of hemoglobin are energetically close to one another. This conclusion is based on several pieces of evidence: The interconversion between high- and low-spin forms is easily accomplished by a change in ligand at the sixth position or by a change in pH or temperature. As examples, ferrihemoglobin hydroxide at room temperature is a mixture of high- and low-spin varieties (GEORGE et al., 1964); Fe^{2+} complexes of the type $Fe^{2+}N_6$ have been observed to cross over from $^5T_2(t_2^4e^2)$ at high temperature to $^1A_1(t_2^6)$ at cryogenic temperatures (KONIG and KREMER, 1971). The detailed evidence, however, is derived from ESR and magnetic susceptibility experiments which are discussed in this chapter.

KOTANI (1968) has pointed out that the ability of hemoglobin to exist in high- or low-spin states confers upon the molecule a degree of electronic flexibility or "softness" which may have significance for its biological function. We shall have occasion to return to this conjecture.

In ferric compounds there is also a $^4T_1$ state (Fig. 5.7) whose energy near the cross-over is comparable to that of $^6A_1$ and $^2T_2$. As in the case of the free ion (Section 5.1) in which ^6S interacts with ^4P through a spin-orbit coupling, there is a similar interaction between $^6A_1$ and $^4T_1$. This turns out to have an important effect on the degeneracy of $^6A_1$, as will be shown in Section 6.3. Furthermore, since $^2T_2$ and $^4T_1$ are coupled by the spin-orbit interaction, it follows that the high-spin $^6A_1$ is coupled, albeit weakly, with the low-spin $^2T_2$ state. Finally, it should be kept in mind that the $(3d)^5$ configuration in ferric compounds is subject to Kramers' theorem. This means that without a magnetic field at least twofold degeneracies will persist no matter how the ligands are arranged.

6.1.2 Paramagnetic Susceptibility

The magnetic moment, μ, of an atom or molecule in the direction of an applied magnetic field, H, is defined by

$$\mu = -\frac{\partial E_n}{\partial H} \tag{6.1.3}$$

where E_n is the energy of the system. To obtain the total magnetic moment per mole, M, it is necessary to perform a statistical average over the thermal distribution of magnetic moments:

$$M = N \frac{\sum\limits_n \mu e^{-E_n/kT}}{\sum\limits_n e^{-E_n/kT}} \tag{6.1.4}$$

in which N is Avogadro's number; the molar susceptibility, χ, is

$$\chi = \frac{M}{H}. \tag{6.1.5}$$

To implement these equations we need to know the dependence of E_n on the magnetic field. If E_n can be expanded as a power series in H,

$$E_n = E_n^{(0)} + H E_n^{(1)} + H^2 E_n^{(2)} + \cdots \tag{6.1.6}$$

then, under the condition that $M \to 0$ as $H \to 0$,

$$\chi = N \frac{\sum\limits_n \left[\frac{(E_n^{(1)})^2}{kT} - 2 E_n^{(2)} \right] e^{-E_n^{(0)}/kT}}{\sum\limits_n e^{-E_n^{(0)}/kT}} \tag{6.1.7}$$

where, in (6.1.7) only the field-independent terms have been retained.

The interaction of a general multiebetron system with a magnetic field is described by the Hamiltonian (5.4.7)

$$\mathcal{H}_m = \beta\, H \cdot (L + 2S),$$ (6.1.8)

which can also be regarded as the defining relation of the magnetic moment operator μ:

$$\mu = \mu_L + \mu_S = -\beta(L + 2S).$$ (6.1.9)

For a system in which

$$\langle 0|L|0\rangle = 0,$$

indicating a complete quenching, or nonexistence, of orbital angular momentum, the Hamiltonian operator (6.1.8) becomes

$$\mathcal{H}_m = 2\beta\, H \cdot S,$$

and

$$\mu = \mu_S.$$

The energy for this case is

$$E_n = 2\beta H_z \langle \psi_n | S_z | \psi_n \rangle = 2\beta H_z E_n^{(1)}$$

in which the z axis has been oriented parallel to the applied field and the index n labels the $2S+1$ degenerate wave functions, ψ_n. The matrix elements are equal to M_s, which assumes the values $S,\ S-1\cdots -S$; since $E_n^{(2)} = E_n^{(0)} = 0$, the susceptibility as given by (6.1.7) becomes

$$\chi = N \frac{(2\beta^2[S^2 + (S-1)^2 + \cdots (-S)^2]}{kT(2S+1)} = \frac{4N\beta^2}{3kT} S(S+1).$$ (6.1.10)

Eq. (6.1.10) is Curie's Law when the magnetic moments are associated entirely with spin alignments. It is convenient to define an effective magnetic moment μ_e, such that

$$\chi = \frac{N\mu_e^2}{3kT}.$$ (6.1.11)

Comparison with (6.1.10) gives

$$\mu_e = 2\beta[S(S+1)]^{\frac{1}{2}}.$$ (6.1.12)

An effective Bohr magneton number, n_e, may be defined by

$$\mu_e = n_e \beta$$

or

$$n_e = 2[S(S+1)]^{\frac{1}{2}}.$$ (6.1.13)

The effective Bohr magneton numbers for several values of S are given in Table 6.1.
    In the free ion the presence of an orbital angular momentum changes (6.1.10) into

$$\chi = N \frac{g^2 \beta^2}{3kT} J(J+1)$$ (6.1.14)

where J is the quantum number of total angular momentum corresponding to the coupling

$$J = L + S$$

Table 6.1. *Effective Bohr magneton numbers*

S	n_e
$\frac{1}{2}$	1.73
1	2.83
$\frac{3}{2}$	3.87
2	4.90
$\frac{5}{2}$	5.92

and g is the Landé g factor or the spectroscopic splitting g factor given by

$$g = \frac{3}{2} + \frac{S(S+1)-L(L+1)}{2J(J+1)}. \tag{6.1.15}$$

Eq. (6.1.14) is analogous to (6.1.10) and is a statement of Curie's Law for the more general case when both orbital and spin angular momenta are present. Also, by analogy with (6.1.13), an effective magnetic moment is given by

$$\mu_e = g\beta[J(J+1)]^{\frac{1}{2}}$$

and an effective Bohr magneton number by

$$n_e = g[J(J+1)]^{\frac{1}{2}}. \tag{6.1.16}$$

The general effect of a crystal field is to remove spatial degeneracies; this tends to quench orbital angular momentum because for an orbital singlet the expectation values of L_x, L_y, and L_z are zero. On the other hand, spin-orbit coupling restores some contribution from orbital angular momentum. When both effects are present the magnetic susceptibility can be expected to depart from the value that would be obtained when spin angular momenta alone are present. This is often described as incomplete quenching.

Experimentally, a measurement of susceptibility includes the diamagnetic contribution, i.e.

$$\chi_{exp} = \chi_{dia} + N\frac{n_e^2\beta^2}{3kT}. \tag{6.1.17}$$

Since the paramagnetic susceptibility is inversely proportional to temperature while the diagamagnetic part is independent of temperature, χ_{dia} may be evaluated by extrapolating the experimental susceptibility to $T = \infty$. We then have

$$n_e = \left[\frac{3k(\chi_{exp}-\chi_{dia})T}{N\beta^2}\right]^{1/2}. \tag{6.1.18}$$

There is a good deal of overlap in the information derived from ESR and that derived from susceptibility measurements. The former focuses on the magnetic properties of the lowest electronic state while the latter depends on the electronic populations in all the levels accessible to electrons at the prevailing temperature. When experiments are conducted over a range of temperature to alter the electronic populations, it is possible to obtain information on the level structure of the first few low-lying states.

6.2 Electron Spin Resonance of Low-Spin Ferrihemoglobin

The ESR spectra of a large number of low-spin hemoglobin derivatives have been examined (PEISACH and BLUMBERG, 1971; BLUMBERG and PEISACH, 1971). They all have the general appearance of Fig. 6.1 and are characterized by three distinct g values in the range of 1 to 3. A good example is ferrihemoglobin azide (Table 6.2), whose principal g values (GIBSON and INGRAM, 1957) are

$$g_x = 1.72, \quad g_y = 2.22 \quad \text{and} \quad g_z = 2.80,$$

where g_x and g_y refer to a magnetic field parallel to the heme plane and g_z to a perpendicular field.

There are essentially two parts to a theoretical interpretation of ESR spectra. The first task is to deduce the properties of the electronic states which give rise to the observed spectra; the second—usually the more difficult task—is to extract information regarding structural features or physical mechanisms. We shall postpone the latter question until Section 6.5.

The g values of low-spin hemoglobins have been analyzed (GRIFFITH, 1957; KOTANI, 1961) on the basis of the hypothesis that the cubic splitting parameter, Δ, is large compared with the pairing energies. This means that the e orbitals are energetically far above the t_2 orbitals, so that all five $3d$ electrons of Fe^{3+} occupy t_2 orbitals. The electronic configuration is therefore t_2^5 and the only possible term is $^2T_2$. From here on, the analysis proceeds on the basis of the t_2 orbitals alone without reference to any excited configurations[6].

Since the t_2 orbitals are 3-fold degenerate, the maximum occupation is six electrons; the five-electron configuration t_2^5 therefore leaves a single hole which, in all important respects, behaves precisely as a single electron. A configuration such as $|\xi^- \eta^2 \zeta^2\rangle$, for example, can be replaced by an equivalent hole described by $|\xi^+\rangle$; this is an important simplification both computationally and conceptually.

We are now led to the following picture: since the g values of hemoglobin azide are all substantially different from the free spin value of 2.0023, the hole does not behave as a free spin. A contribution from orbital angular momentum must be present. From the fact that the principal g values are all different, i.e. $g_x \neq g_y \neq g_z$, it follows that the symmetry at the position of the iron atom must be lower than cubic and in fact lower than tetragonal. It is reasonable to assume rhombic D_2 (or C_{2v}) symmetry. This means that there are three types of crystal field potentials in the Hamiltonian which are, respectively, invariant under the operations of the groups O, D_4 (or C_{4v}) and D_2 (or C_{2v}). Under O, the t_2 orbitals

---

[6]   A more recent discussion by GRIFFITH (1971) indicates that among the large number of spectra observed by PEISACH and BLUMBERG (1971) there are some whose interpretation is improved by invoking configuration interaction between t_2^5 and $t_2^4 e$.

Table 6.2. *Experimental data on magnetic properties of hemoglobin and myoglobin derivatives*

Compound	g	Ref.	$D(\text{cm}^{-1})$	Ref.	$\dfrac{|E|}{D}$	Ref.	n_e [a]	pH	Ref.	Remarks
Methemoglobin	2 6	G1	10.5	B			5.65	6.36	S	
Ferrihemoglobin Hydroxide							4.66	9.73	S	
Ferrihemoglobin Azide	1.72 2.22 2.80	G2					2.35	6.72	S	
Ferrihemoglobin Cyanide							2.50	6.72	S	
Ferrihemoglobin Fluoride		B	6.3 ±0.12				5.76	7.10	S	Resonance lines are split due to interaction with ^{19}F nucleus (PE)
Deoxyhemoglobin							5.4		P	
Metmyoglobin	2 6	G1	9.5 ±1.5	B	$\frac{1}{400}$	K	5.73	6.44	S	
Ferrimyoglobin Hydroxide							5.04	11.60	S	
Ferrimyoglobin Azide	1.72 2.22 2.80	G2					3.30	6.80	S	
Ferrimyoglobin Cyanide							1.96	7.41	S	
Ferrimyoglobin Fluoride	2 6		5.94 ±0.08	B	$\frac{3}{800}$	K	5.77	6.84	S	Resonance lines are split due to interaction with ^{19}F nucleus (M, PE)

G1 GIBSON *et al.* (1958)   S   SCHELER *et al.* (1957);   K KOTANI and MORIMOTO (1967)
G2 GIBSON and INGRAM (1957)   SMITH and WILLIAMS (1970)   M MORIMOTO and KOTANI (1966)
B   BRACKETT *et al.* (1971)   P   PAULING and CORYELL (1936)   PE PEISACH *et al.* (1971)

[a] All data at 293°K.

ξ, η, ζ (or d_{yz}, d_{zx}, d_{xy}) are degenerate; reduction of the symmetry to D_4 (or C_{4v}) separates the ζ orbital from ξ and η, which still remain degenerate. Further reduction of the symmetry to D_2 (or C_{2v}) separates the ξ and η orbitals, thereby lifting the orbital degeneracy completely. Thus, under the influence of the low-symmetry environment, ξ, η, ζ are each orbital singlets with energies ε_ξ, ε_η and ε_ζ respectively, as shown in Fig. 5.5. Each orbital still has a 2-fold spin degeneracy which, according to Kramers' theorem, cannot be removed by any combination of electric fields. We must also include spin-orbit coupling to allow for possible mixing of the orbitals. The final result will then be a set of Kramers doublets expressed as linear combinations of the ξ, η, ζ orbitals (including spin) and the origin of the observed ESR spectra will be attributed to transitions between magnetic substates of the Kramers doublets.

Examination of the matrix in Table 5.13 reveals that ξ^+, η^+, and ζ^- have nonvanishing spin-orbit coupling matrix elements among themselves, and the situation is similar in the set ξ^-, η^- and ζ^+. Matrix elements of orbitals from one set with orbitals from the other vanish. The general structure of the Kramers doublet will therefore be

$$\psi^+ = a_1 \xi^+ + b_1 \eta^+ + c_1 \zeta^- ,$$
$$\psi^- = a_2 \xi^- + b_2 \eta^- + c_2 \zeta^+ .$$

Although there appear to be six constants, they are not all independent because ψ_1 and ψ_2 must be related by the Kramers operator i.e. $\psi_2 = K\psi_1$. The lowest Kramers doublet may therefore be written

$$\psi_1^+ = A_1 \xi^+ + iB_1 \eta^+ + C_1 \zeta^- ,$$
$$\psi_1^- = -A_1 \xi^- + iB_1 \eta^- + C_1 \zeta^+ ,$$

(6.2.1)

in which the coefficients A_1, B_1 and C_1 are taken to be real (KOTANI, 1961).

Table 6.3. *Matrices of* $\mathbf{l} + 2\mathbf{s}$ *for the lowest Kramers doublet*

$l_z + 2s_z$	ψ_1^+	ψ_1^-	
ψ_1^+	$(A_1 - B_1)^2 - C_1^2$	0	
ψ_1^-	0	$-[(A_1 - B_1)^2 - C_1^2]$	a)
$l_x + 2s_x$	ψ_1^+	ψ_1^-	
ψ_1^+	0	$(B_1 + C_1)^2 - A_1^2$	
ψ_1^-	$(B_1 + C_1)^2 - A_1^2$	0	b)
$l_y + 2s_y$	ψ_1^+	ψ_1^-	
ψ_1^+	0	$i[(A_1 - C_1)^2 - B_1^2]$	
ψ_1^-	$-i[(A_1 - C_1)^2 - B_1^2]$	0	c)

In order to interpret the g values associated with ESR experiments, it is necessary to obtain the eigenvalues of the magnetic interaction Hamiltonian (5.4.7). With the help of Table 5.16 it is possible to construct the matrices of $\mathbf{l} + 2\mathbf{s}$ in the basis set ψ_1^+, ψ_1^-. These are given in Table 6.3. For a magnetic field in the z direction, the eigenvalues are

$$E_+^{(z)} = \beta H_z [(A_1 - B_1)^2 - C_1^2],$$
$$E_-^{(z)} = -\beta H_z [(A_1 - B_1)^2 - C_1^2],$$

(6.2.2)

indicating that the two-fold degeneracy of the doublet is lifted by the magnetic field. The separation in energy of the two components of the doublet is

$$\Delta E = E_+^{(z)} - E_-^{(z)} = 2\beta H_z[(A_1 - B_1)^2 - C_1^2] \tag{6.2.3}$$

and electron-spin resonance will be observed when the electromagnetic energy satisfies the condition

$$\hbar\omega = g_z \beta H_z = \Delta E \tag{6.2.4}$$

or

$$g_z = 2|(A_1 - B_1)^2 - C_1^2| . \tag{6.2.5}$$

The eigenvalues of $l_x + 2s_x$ and $l_y + 2s_y$ are obtained from the solution of the secular determinant associated with the corresponding matrices in Table 6.3. They are

$$E^{(x)} = \pm\beta H_x[(B_1 + C_1)^2 - A_1^2],$$
$$E^{(y)} = \pm\beta H_y[(A_1 - C_1)^2 - B_1^2]. \tag{6.2.6}$$

Therefore the principal components of the g tensor are

$$g_x = 2|(B_1 + C_1)^2 - A_1^2|,$$
$$g_y = 2|(A_1 - C_1)^2 - B_1^2|, \tag{6.2.7}$$
$$g_z = 2|(A_1 - B_1)^2 - C_1^2|,$$

where absolute values are used to ensure that g_x, g_y and g_z are positive quantities.

An additional condition is that each Kramers doublet be normalized or that

$$A_1^2 + B_1^2 + C_1^2 = 1 . \tag{6.2.8}$$

The three relations contained in (6.2.7) together with the normalization condition provide us with four equations for the three unknown coefficients A_1, B_1, C_1. It then becomes a matter of optimizing the coefficients so as to give the best fit with experimental g values. KOTANI's (1961) values are

$$A_1 = 0.973, \quad B_1 = -0.209, \quad C_1 = -0.097 . \tag{6.2.9}$$

It is assumed, and borne out by subsequent calculation, that the observed g values are associated with the splitting of the lowest Kramers doublet which, with (6.2.1), is given by

$$\psi_1^+ = 0.973\,\xi^+ - 0.209\,i\eta^+ - 0.097\,\zeta^- ,$$
$$\psi_1^- = -0.973\,\xi^- - 0.209\,i\eta^- - 0.097\,\zeta^+ . \tag{6.2.10}$$

We note that the coefficient of ξ^+ in ψ_1^+ (or the coefficient of ξ^- in ψ_1^-) has an absolute value close to unity so that the lowest Kramers doublet closely resembles the ξ orbital. Nevertheless, the terms in η and ζ, whose presence is directly associated with the spin-orbit interaction, exert an important effect on the g values.

It is now possible to calculate the energy of the orbitals, ξ, η, ζ. For this purpose let the combined Hamiltonian of the spin-orbit coupling and the crystal field, V, be

$$\mathcal{H} = -\lambda\,\mathbf{l}\cdot\mathbf{s} + V \tag{6.2.11}$$

where we have used $\lambda(>0)$ as the spin-orbit coupling parameter in place of ζ (5.1.4) to avoid confusion with the ζ orbital. The negative sign in the first term of (6.2.11) comes about because the system under discussion is described by a hole which carries an equivalent positive charge. We assume $\xi, \eta,$ and ζ are eigenfunctions of V with eigenvalues $\varepsilon_\xi, \varepsilon_\eta, \varepsilon_\zeta$. Then the condition

$$\mathscr{H} \psi_1^+ = E \psi_1^+ , \qquad (6.2.12)$$

where ψ_1^+ is given by (6.2.1), leads to a set of relations between the orbital energies and the coefficients A_1, B_1, C_1. This can be seen by multiplying (6.2.12) on the left by ξ^+, η^+, ζ^- respectively, and evaluating the resulting matrix elements with the help of Table 5.13. We then get

$$A_1(\varepsilon_\xi - E) - (i B_1)\frac{i}{2}\lambda + C_1\frac{\lambda}{2} = 0 ,$$

$$A_1 \frac{i}{2}\lambda + (i B_1)(\varepsilon_\eta - E) - C_1\frac{i}{2}\lambda = 0 , \qquad (6.2.13)$$

$$A_1 \frac{\lambda}{2} + (i B_1)\frac{i}{2}\lambda + C_1(\varepsilon_\zeta - E) = 0 .$$

A_1, B_1, C_1 are the coefficients in the lowest Kramers doublet given by (6.2.9) and E is the energy of the doublet. We can set $E=0$ (or any other arbitrarily chosen energy) since differences in energy are all that matter. Thus

$$\varepsilon_\xi = -\left[\frac{B_1 + C_1}{A_1}\right]\frac{\lambda}{2} = 0.157\,\lambda ,$$

$$\varepsilon_\eta = \left[\frac{C_1 - A_1}{B_1}\right]\frac{\lambda}{2} = 2.56\,\lambda , \qquad (6.2.14)$$

$$\varepsilon_\zeta = \left[\frac{B_1 - A_1}{C_1}\right]\frac{\lambda}{2} = 6.09\,\lambda$$

and

$$\text{(hole)} \qquad \begin{aligned} \varepsilon_\xi - \varepsilon_\eta &= -2.403\,\lambda , \\ \varepsilon_\xi - \varepsilon_\zeta &= -5.936\,\lambda . \end{aligned} \qquad (6.2.15)$$

At this stage of the calculation, the coefficients which describe the lowest Kramers doublet and the orbital separations associated with the single hole are known. As a final step we compute the coefficients describing the remaining two doublets. Let the general doublet be described as in (6.2.1)

$$\begin{aligned} \psi^+ &= A\xi^+ + i B\eta^+ + C\zeta^- \\ \psi^- &= -A\xi^- + i B\eta^- + C\zeta^+ . \end{aligned} \qquad (6.2.16)$$

As before, the Hamiltonian (6.2.11) and the condition

$$\mathscr{H} \psi^+ = E \psi^+$$

lead to secular equations of the form of (6.2.13) with arbitrary coefficients A, B, C.

The condition for the existence of solutions is the vanishing of the secular determinant:

$$\begin{vmatrix} \varepsilon_\xi - E & -\dfrac{i}{2}\lambda & \dfrac{\lambda}{2} \\[2ex] \dfrac{i}{2}\lambda & \varepsilon_\eta - E & -\dfrac{i}{2}\lambda \\[2ex] \dfrac{\lambda}{2} & \dfrac{i}{2}\lambda & \varepsilon_\zeta - E \end{vmatrix} = 0. \tag{6.2.17}$$

The three roots of the secular determinant are the energies of the three Kramers doublets. Since ε_ξ, ε_η, and ε_ζ are known from (6.2.14), the secular determinant may be solved in terms of λ. Each root, when substituted into the secular equations will yield a set of coefficients for that particular doublet. The final results as given by KOTANI (1961) are

k	Excitation E	A_k	B_k	C_k	
1	0	0.973	−0.209	−0.097	(6.2.18)
2	2.613λ	0.219	0.970	0.108	
3	6.200λ	0.071	−0.126	0.990	

We note that each of the Kramers doublets corresponds very closely to one of the orbitals ξ, η, ζ.

From (6.2.14) it is seen that the ξ orbital lies lowest in energy, with the η and ζ orbitals lying above in that order. It is necessary to emphasize once again that these orbital energies refer to a single hole which is complementary to the five-electron system. If the hole were to be replaced by an electron, the orbital energies would be reversed in sign and in place of (6.2.15) we should have

$$\text{(electron)} \qquad \begin{aligned} \varepsilon_\zeta - \varepsilon_\eta &= 2.403\,\lambda, \\ \varepsilon_\zeta - \varepsilon_\xi &= 5.936\,\lambda. \end{aligned} \tag{6.2.19}$$

With λ approximately equal to $435\ \text{cm}^{-1}$, the orbital separations are $\varepsilon_\zeta - \varepsilon_\eta = 1040\ \text{cm}^{-1}$ and $\varepsilon_\zeta - \varepsilon_\xi = 2580\ \text{cm}^{-1}$. The tetragonal splitting (δ) and the rhombic splitting (μ) are

$$\begin{aligned} \delta &= (\varepsilon_\zeta - \varepsilon_\xi) - \tfrac{1}{2}(\varepsilon_\zeta - \varepsilon_\eta) = 4.73\,\lambda \\ &= 2060\ \text{cm}^{-1}, \\[1ex] \mu &= \varepsilon_\zeta - \varepsilon_\eta = 2.40\,\lambda \\ &= 1040\ \text{cm}^{-1} \end{aligned} \tag{6.2.20}$$

with the ζ-orbital lying lowest as shown in Fig. 6.3. It is likely that in hemoglobin, as in other complexes, λ is somewhat less than $435\ \text{cm}^{-1}$ which is the free ion value for Fe^{3+}; the numerical values in (6.2.20) are therefore likely to be too high. Nevertheless, the orbitals are so far apart that at cryogenic temperatures—or even at room temperature—there is essentially no electronic population in the upper two doublets; only the lowest one is occupied and it is the only one, as stated previously, that contributes to the ESR spectrum.

$$\begin{array}{ccc}
\rule{2cm}{0.4pt}\; \xi\;(d_{yz}) & & \rule{2cm}{0.4pt}\;3 \\
\quad 2.40\,\lambda & & \quad 3.59\,\lambda \\
\rule{2cm}{0.4pt}\;\eta\;(d_{zx}) & & \\
\delta = 4.73\,\lambda & & \rule{2cm}{0.4pt}\;2 \\
\quad 3.53\,\lambda & & \quad 2.61\,\lambda \\
\rule{2cm}{0.4pt}\;\zeta\;(d_{xy}) & & \rule{2cm}{0.4pt}\;1 \\
(a) & & (b)
\end{array}$$

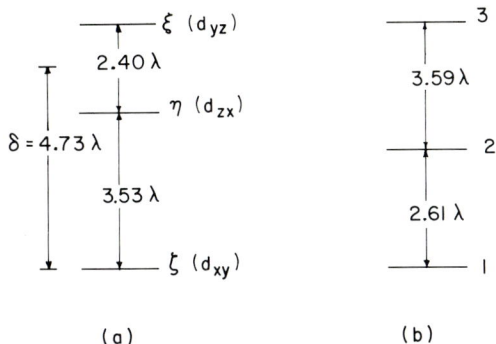

Fig. 6.3 a and b. a) One-electron orbital energies, b) Kramer's doublets. λ is the spin-orbit coupling parameter ($\sim 435\ \mathrm{cm}^{-1}$), δ is the tetragonal splitting

The form of the Kramers doublets given in (6.2.1) is not unique. GRIFFITH (1957) worked with the basis set $|t_2 1\rangle, |t_2 0\rangle, |t_2 -1\rangle$ which are related to the ξ, η, ζ orbitals as shown in Table 5.5. The procedure is entirely analogous to that described above, though of course, the coefficients will be quite different[7]. The g values of a large number of low-spin ferric hemoproteins have been analyzed by HARRIS-LOEW (1970).

6.3 Electron Spin Resonance of High-Spin Ferrihemoglobin

In contrast to low-spin ferrihemoglobins whose ESR spectra have three g values and all three signals are of comparable magnitude, the spectra of most high-spin ferrihemoglobins (Table 6.2) show only two resonances: a strong one at $g_x = g_y = g_\perp = 6$ and a much weaker one at $g_z = g_{\parallel} = 2$ (Fig. 6.2). Parallel and perpendicular refer to the 4-fold-symmetry axis or z axis, which is perpendicular to the heme plane (Fig. 2.1).

We have seen that a ferric ion with an electronic configuration described by $(3d)^5$ gives rise to a ^6S ground state. The application of an octahedral crystal field or, indeed, a field of lower symmetry, produces no splitting; the ground state remains 6-fold degenerate. The application of a magnetic field, with or without a crystal field, lifts the 6-fold degeneracy and produces a set of equally spaced levels with a separation of $2\beta H$. The selection rule $\Delta M_S = \pm 1$ permits transitions only between adjacent levels resulting in $g = 2$, regardless of the orientation of the magnetic field. Such an isotropic value of g is clearly contradictory to the experimental facts.

As in the previous discussion of low-spin hemoglobin, it will be necessary to invoke spin-orbit coupling. However, it is immediately recognized that there are no first-order effects, i.e. no spin-orbit coupling among the substates of $^6A_1$.

[7] KOTANI (1961) and GRIFFITH (1957) also treat the numerical data differently. For δ and μ, GRIFFITH obtained 3.32 λ and 2.26 λ, respectively, in place of the values shown in (6.2.20) which correspond to KOTANI's values.

Lowering the symmetry does not alter the situation; it is therefore necessary to carry the calculation to a higher order to permit excited states to interact with the ground state. We have seen that in the free ion (Section 5.1), ^6S couples with ^4P. When the symmetry is lowered to O, ^6S and ^4P become $^6A_1$ and $^4T_1$ respectively; it is therefore to be expected that the latter two states will interact by spin-orbit coupling. The notion that this interaction may have a significant effect on $^6A_1$ becomes all the more plausible when it is recalled (Section 5.5) that in hemoglobin $\Delta \approx \Delta_c$ and that in this region the configurations $t_2^3 e^2 \, {}^6A_1$ and $t_2^4 e \, {}^4T_1$ (as well as $t_2^5 \, {}^2T_2$) are energetically close to one another.

6.3.1 Spin-Orbit Coupling

The first task, then, is to compute the matrix elements of the spin-orbit coupling operator (5.1.4) between $t_2^3 e^2 \, {}^6A_1$ and $t_2^4 e \, {}^4T_1$—more specifically, as discussed in Section 5.5—between $t_2^3 ({}^4A_2) e^2 ({}^3A_2) \, {}^6A_1$ and $t_2^4 ({}^3T_1) e ({}^2E) \, {}^4T_1$. In the case of low-spin hemoglobin it was possible to replace the t_2^5 configuration by a single hole. This simplified the calculation considerably; in the present case such a stratagem is not possible and it is necessary to work with the 5-electron system. Fortunately, general methods have been developed in close analogy with those employed for free ions (Section 5.1). These are based on Racah's formalism, which was originally developed for atomic systems and subsequently extended to low-symmetry groups appropriate for the description of molecules. GRIFFITH (1962) gives a detailed treatment of these methods. His expression for the spin-orbit coupling matrix element (in units of the spin-orbit coupling parameter) is the following:

$$\langle S\,h\,M\,\theta | \mathcal{H}_s | S'\,h'\,M'\,\theta' \rangle = \langle S\,h \| \mathcal{H}_s \| S'\,h' \rangle \sum_i (-1)^{i+1+S-M} [-1]^{h+\theta}$$

$$\times \bar{V} \begin{pmatrix} S & S' & 1 \\ -M & M' & i \end{pmatrix} V \begin{pmatrix} h & h' & T_1 \\ -\theta & \theta' & -i \end{pmatrix}. \tag{6.3.1}$$

S and S' are the spins of the initial and final states respectively, and h and h' are the representations of the initial and final states respectively. In the cubic group O, h and h' may each stand for A_1, A_2, E_1, T_1 or T_2.

M and M' are the projection quantum numbers of S and S' respectively, i.e. M takes on the values $S, S-1 \cdots -S$.

θ and θ' are components of the representations h and h' respectively, $\mathcal{H}_s$ is the spin-orbit coupling operator.

i is a number which takes on the values $1, 0$ or -1. $[-1]^{h+\theta}$ is a special symbol with the following meaning:

$$[-1]^{h+\theta} = [-1]^h [-1]^\theta$$

when h is A_1, A_2 or E, $[-1]^h = 1$,
when θ is a component of A_1, A_2 or E, $[-1]^\theta = 1$,
when h is T_1 or T_2, $[-1]^h = -1$,
when θ is a component of T_1, $[-1]^\theta = -1$,
when θ is a component of T_2, $[-1]^\theta = 1$.

$\bar{V}\begin{pmatrix} S & S' & 1 \\ -M & M' & i \end{pmatrix}$ is a 3-j symbol. It differs from the 3-j symbol defined by

ROTENBERG et al. (1959) by a phase factor. The relation between the two is

$$\bar{V}\begin{pmatrix} S & S' & 1 \\ -M & M' & i \end{pmatrix} = (-1)^{S+S'+1}\begin{pmatrix} S & S' & 1 \\ -M & M' & i \end{pmatrix}. \tag{6.3.2}$$

$V\begin{pmatrix} h & h' & T_1 \\ -\theta & \theta' & -i \end{pmatrix}$ is a low-symmetry coupling coefficient. GRIFFITH (1962) gives

tabulations for the cubic group, and again, the lack of universality in regard to phase conventions should be borne in mind.

$\langle Sh\|\mathcal{H}_s\|S'h'\rangle$ is a reduced matrix element; it is independent of M and θ. The specific expressions for the reduced matrix element depend on the electronic configurations. For d electrons, the reduced matrix element, when taken between a term belonging to a configuration $t_2^{m-1}e^n$ and a term belonging to $t_2^m e^{n-1}$, is given by

$$\langle t_2^{m-1}(S_1 h_1)e^n(S_2 h_2)Sh\|\mathcal{H}_s\|t_2^m(S_1' h_1')e^{n-1}(S_2' h_2')S'h'\rangle$$
$$= (-1)^{S_1-S_1'-S_2+S_2'+h_1+h_1'+h_2+h_2'}$$
$$\times [mn(2S+1)(2S'+1)(2S_1'+1)(2S_2+1)\lambda(h)\lambda(h')\lambda(h_1')\lambda(h_2)]^{\frac{1}{2}}$$
$$\times \langle t_2^{m-1}(S_1 h_1), t_2|\} t_2^m S_1' h_1'\rangle\langle e^n S_2 h_2\{|e, e^{n-1}(S_2' h_2')\rangle \tag{6.3.3}$$
$$\times \bar{X}\begin{bmatrix} S_1 & S_2 & S \\ S_1' & S_2' & S' \\ \frac{1}{2} & \frac{1}{2} & 1 \end{bmatrix} X\begin{bmatrix} h_1 & h_2 & h \\ h_1' & h_2' & h' \\ t_2 & e & T_1 \end{bmatrix}\langle \tfrac{1}{2}e\|su\|\tfrac{1}{2}t_2\rangle.$$

In Eq. (6.3.3), S and h are the spin and representation respectively of a term such as $^6A_1$ or $^4T_1$. S_1, h_1 and S_2, h_2 are spins and representations arising from the electron configurations t_2^{m-1} and e^n respectively. It is understood that S_1 and S_2 are coupled together to form S while h_1 and h_2 are coupled to form h. In the same way, S_1' and S_2' give rise to S'; h_1' and h_2' to h'.

The symbol $(-1)^h$ is defined by

$$(-1)^{A_1} = (-1)^E = (-1)^{T_2} = +1,$$
$$(-1)^{A_2} = (-1)^{T_1} = -1. \tag{6.3.4}$$

$\lambda(h)$ and $\lambda(h')$ are the degrees of representations h and h' respectively, e.g. $\lambda(A_1) = 1$, $\lambda(A_2) = 1$, $\lambda(E) = 2$, $\lambda(T_1) = 3$, $\lambda(T_2) = 3$.

The quantities $\langle t_2^{m-1}(S_1 h_1), t_2|\} t_2^m S_1' h_1'\rangle$ and $\langle e^n S_2 h_2\{|e, e^{n-1}(S_2' h_2')\rangle$ are fractional parentage coefficients whose definition with respect to the low symmetry groups is analogous to (5.1.3). $\bar{X}$ is a 9-j symbol (ROTENBERG et al., 1959) and X is its low-symmetry analog. Finally, $\langle \tfrac{1}{2}e\|su\|\tfrac{1}{2}t_2\rangle$ is a one-electron reduced matrix element of the spin-orbit coupling operator (GRIFFITH, 1962). Let us now illustrate the application of (6.3.3) to the calculation of the reduced matrix element between $^6A_1$ and $^4T_1$.

The lowest energy $^4T_1$ term originates from the configuration $t_2^4(^3T_1)e(^2E)$ as discussed in Section 5.5; similarly $^6A_1$ must come from $t_2^3(^4A_2)e^2(^3A_2)$. The reduced matrix element (6.3.3) then becomes

$$M = \langle t_2^3(^4A_2)e^2(^3A_2)^6A_1\|\mathcal{H}_s\|t_2^4(^3T_1)e(^2E)^4T_1\rangle, \tag{6.3.5}$$

in which

$$S_1 = \tfrac{3}{2}, \qquad S_2 = 1, \qquad S = \tfrac{5}{2},$$
$$S_1' = 1, \qquad S_2' = \tfrac{1}{2}, \qquad S' = \tfrac{3}{2},$$
$$h_1 = A_2, \qquad h_2 = A_2, \qquad h = A_1,$$
$$h_1' = T_1, \qquad h_2' = E, \qquad h' = T_1,$$

$$(-1)^{S_1 - S_1' - S_2 + S_2' + h_1 + h_1' + h_2 + h_2'} = (-1)^{\frac{3}{2} - 1 - 1 + \frac{1}{2} + A_2 + T_1 + A_2 + E} = -1,$$

$$[mn(2S+1)(2S'+1)(2S_1'+1)(2S_2+1)\lambda(h)\lambda(h')\lambda(h_1')\lambda(h_2)]^{\frac{1}{2}}$$
$$= [4 \cdot 2 \cdot 6 \cdot 4 \cdot 3 \cdot 3 \cdot 1 \cdot 3 \cdot 3 \cdot 1]^{\frac{1}{2}} = 72\sqrt{3},$$

$$\langle t_2^{m-1}(S_1 h_1), t_2 | \} t_2^m S_1' h_1' \rangle = \langle t_2^3 (^4 A_2), t_2 | \} t_2^4 (^3 T_1) \rangle = -\frac{1}{\sqrt{3}},$$

$$\langle e^n S_2 h_2 \{| e, e^{n-1}(S_2' h_2') \rangle = \langle e^2 (^3 A_2) \{| e, e(^2 E) \rangle = 1,$$

$$\bar{X} \begin{bmatrix} S_1 & S_2 & S \\ S_1' & S_2' & S' \\ \tfrac{1}{2} & \tfrac{1}{2} & 1 \end{bmatrix} = \bar{X} \begin{bmatrix} \tfrac{3}{2} & 1 & \tfrac{5}{2} \\ 1 & \tfrac{1}{2} & \tfrac{3}{2} \\ \tfrac{1}{2} & \tfrac{1}{2} & 1 \end{bmatrix}.$$

The $\bar{X}$ coefficients (9-j symbols) are expressible in terms of 6-j symbols (Rotenberg *et al.*, 1959):

$$\bar{X} \begin{bmatrix} \tfrac{3}{2} & 1 & \tfrac{5}{2} \\ 1 & \tfrac{1}{2} & \tfrac{3}{2} \\ \tfrac{1}{2} & \tfrac{1}{2} & 1 \end{bmatrix} = \begin{bmatrix} \tfrac{3}{2} & 1 & \tfrac{5}{2} \\ 1 & \tfrac{1}{2} & \tfrac{3}{2} \\ \tfrac{1}{2} & \tfrac{1}{2} & 1 \end{bmatrix}$$

$$= \sum_j (-1)^{2j}(2j+1) \begin{Bmatrix} \tfrac{3}{2} & 1 & \tfrac{1}{2} \\ \tfrac{1}{2} & 1 & j \end{Bmatrix} \begin{Bmatrix} 1 & \tfrac{1}{2} & \tfrac{1}{2} \\ 1 & j & \tfrac{3}{2} \end{Bmatrix} \begin{Bmatrix} \tfrac{5}{2} & \tfrac{3}{2} & 1 \\ j & \tfrac{3}{2} & 1 \end{Bmatrix}. \qquad (6.3.6)$$

In the general 6-j symbol $\begin{Bmatrix} j_1 & j_2 & j_3 \\ l_1 & l_2 & l_3 \end{Bmatrix}$ it is necessary for $(j_1 j_2 j_3)$, $(l_1 l_2 j_3)$, $(j_1 l_2 l_3)$ and $(l_1 j_2 l_3)$ to form triangles; for example $(j_1 j_2 j_3)$ forms a triangle when

$$j_1 + j_2 - j_3 \geqslant 0; \qquad j_1 - j_2 + j_3 \geqslant 0; \qquad -j_1 + j_2 + j_3 \geqslant 0 \qquad (6.3.7)$$

and

$$j_1 + j_2 + j_3 \text{ is an integer}.$$

The j values over which we need to sum are those that result in nonvanishing 6-j symbols. For

$$\begin{Bmatrix} \tfrac{3}{2} & 1 & \tfrac{1}{2} \\ \tfrac{1}{2} & 1 & j \end{Bmatrix} \neq 0$$

it is necessary for $(\tfrac{3}{2}\ 1\ j)$ and $(\tfrac{1}{2}\ 1\ j)$ to form triangles. The first case is satisfied by $j = \tfrac{1}{2}, \tfrac{3}{2}, \tfrac{5}{2}$ and the second case by $j = \tfrac{1}{2}, \tfrac{3}{2}$. Hence we obtain nonzero values of the 6-j symbol only when $j = \tfrac{1}{2}$ or $\tfrac{3}{2}$. When $j = \tfrac{5}{2}$, the second triad, $(\tfrac{1}{2}\ 1\ j)$, cannot form a triangle and the 6-j symbol vanishes. The second 6-j symbol can be rearranged so as to become identical to the first; the third 6-j symbol has nonzero values for $j = \tfrac{1}{2}, \tfrac{3}{2}, \tfrac{5}{2}$. The summation therefore extends over two values of j, namely $\tfrac{1}{2}$ and $\tfrac{3}{2}$.

From a table of 6-j coefficients we find

$j = \frac{1}{2}$,

$$\begin{Bmatrix} \frac{3}{2} & 1 & \frac{1}{2} \\ \frac{1}{2} & 1 & \frac{1}{2} \end{Bmatrix} = \begin{Bmatrix} 1 & \frac{1}{2} & \frac{1}{2} \\ 1 & \frac{1}{2} & \frac{3}{2} \end{Bmatrix} = -\frac{1}{3},$$

$$\begin{Bmatrix} \frac{5}{2} & \frac{3}{2} & 1 \\ \frac{1}{2} & \frac{3}{2} & 1 \end{Bmatrix} = -\frac{1}{4},$$

$j = \frac{3}{2}$,

$$\begin{Bmatrix} \frac{3}{2} & 1 & \frac{1}{2} \\ \frac{1}{2} & 1 & \frac{3}{2} \end{Bmatrix} = \begin{Bmatrix} 1 & \frac{1}{2} & \frac{1}{2} \\ 1 & \frac{3}{2} & \frac{3}{2} \end{Bmatrix} = \frac{1}{6}(\frac{5}{2})^{\frac{1}{2}}.$$

Therefore

$$\bar{X} = (-1)^1 \cdot 2 \cdot -\frac{1}{3} \cdot -\frac{1}{3} \cdot -\frac{1}{4} + (-1)^3 \cdot 4 \cdot \frac{1}{6}(\frac{5}{2})^{\frac{1}{2}} \cdot \frac{1}{6}(\frac{5}{2})^{\frac{1}{2}} \cdot -\frac{1}{10} = \frac{1}{18} + \frac{1}{36} = \frac{1}{12}. \quad (6.3.8)$$

$$X \begin{bmatrix} h_1 & h_2 & h \\ h'_1 & h'_2 & h' \\ t_2 & e & T_1 \end{bmatrix} = X \begin{bmatrix} A_2 & A_2 & A_1 \\ T_1 & E & T_1 \\ T_2 & E & T_1 \end{bmatrix} = X \begin{bmatrix} T_1 & E & T_1 \\ T_2 & E & T_1 \\ A_2 & A_2 & A_1 \end{bmatrix}.$$

The last form is obtained by interchanging rows according to the symmetry properties of the X coefficients. When an X coefficient contains an A_1 it reduces to a W coefficient according to

$$X \begin{bmatrix} a & b & c \\ d & h & f \\ g & h & A_1 \end{bmatrix} = (-1)^{b+d+f+h} \lambda(c)^{-\frac{1}{2}} \lambda(g)^{-\frac{1}{2}} \delta_{cf} \delta_{gh} W \begin{pmatrix} a & b & c \\ e & d & g \end{pmatrix}.$$

Therefore

$$X \begin{bmatrix} T_1 & E & T_1 \\ T_2 & E & T_1 \\ A_2 & A_2 & A_1 \end{bmatrix} = (-1)^{E+T_2+T_1+A_2} \lambda(T_1)^{-\frac{1}{2}} \lambda(A_2)^{-\frac{1}{2}} W \begin{pmatrix} T_1 & E & T_1 \\ E & T_2 & A_2 \end{pmatrix}$$

$$= \frac{1}{\sqrt{3}} \cdot -\frac{1}{\sqrt{6}} = -\frac{1}{3} \sqrt{\frac{1}{2}}. \qquad (6.3.9)$$

From Table 10.2 in Griffith (1962),

$$\langle \tfrac{1}{2} e \| s u \| \tfrac{1}{2} t_2 \rangle = -3\sqrt{2}. \qquad (6.3.10)$$

Therefore (6.3.5) becomes

$$M = -1 \cdot 72 \sqrt{3} \cdot -\frac{1}{\sqrt{3}} \cdot \frac{1}{12} \cdot -\frac{1}{3} \sqrt{\frac{1}{2}} \cdot -3\sqrt{2} = 6. \qquad (6.3.11)$$

The matrix elements of spin-orbit coupling between $^6A_1$ and $^4T_1$ are now readily calculated with the aid of Griffith's table of V coefficients and a table of 3-j symbols. The results are listed in Table 6.4. For some purposes it is more convenient to have matrix elements between $^6A_1$ and the rectangular components of $^4T_1$. These are given in Table 6.5 where we have used the relations for the $^4T_1$ components as shown in Table 5.5. More complete tables of matrix elements are given by Griffith (1962) and Weissbluth (1967).

Table 6.5. *Matrix elements of spin-orbit coupling among components of* $^6A_1$ *and (rectangular) components of* $^4T_1$ *(in units of ζ)*

$^6A_1$ \ $^4T_1$	$\frac{3}{2}x$	$\frac{3}{2}y$	$\frac{3}{2}z$	$\frac{1}{2}x$	$\frac{1}{2}y$	$\frac{1}{2}z$	$-\frac{1}{2}x$	$-\frac{1}{2}y$	$-\frac{1}{2}z$	$-\frac{3}{2}x$	$-\frac{3}{2}y$	$-\frac{3}{2}z$
$\frac{5}{2}$	$-i$	-1										
$\frac{3}{2}$			$i\dfrac{2}{\sqrt5}$	$-i\left(\dfrac{3}{5}\right)^{\frac12}$	$-\left(\dfrac{3}{5}\right)^{\frac12}$							
$\frac{1}{2}$	$i\left(\dfrac{1}{10}\right)^{\frac12}$	$-\left(\dfrac{1}{10}\right)^{\frac12}$				$i\left(\dfrac{6}{5}\right)^{\frac12}$	$-i\left(\dfrac{3}{10}\right)^{\frac12}$	$-\left(\dfrac{3}{10}\right)^{\frac12}$				
$-\frac{1}{2}$				$i\left(\dfrac{3}{10}\right)^{\frac12}$	$-\left(\dfrac{3}{10}\right)^{\frac12}$				$i\left(\dfrac{6}{5}\right)^{\frac12}$	$-i\left(\dfrac{1}{10}\right)^{\frac12}$	$-\left(\dfrac{1}{10}\right)^{\frac12}$	
$-\frac{3}{2}$							$i\left(\dfrac{3}{5}\right)^{\frac12}$	$-\left(\dfrac{3}{5}\right)^{\frac12}$				$i\dfrac{2}{\sqrt5}$
$-\frac{5}{2}$										i	-1	

Table 6.4. *Matrix elements of spin-orbit coupling among components of* $^6A_1$ *and (spherical) components of* $^4T_1$ *(in units of* ζ*)*

		$^4T_1\,\frac{1}{2}\,0$	$^4T_1\,-\frac{1}{2}\,1$	$^4T_1\,\frac{3}{2}\,-1$	$^4T_1\,-\frac{3}{2}\,0$	$^4T_1\,\frac{3}{2}\,1$	$^4T_1\,-\frac{1}{2}\,-1$
		$^4T_1\,-\frac{1}{2}\,0$	$^4T_1\,\frac{1}{2}\,-1$	$^4T_1\,-\frac{3}{2}\,1$	$^4T_1\,\frac{3}{2}\,0$	$^4T_1\,-\frac{3}{2}\,-1$	$^4T_1\,\frac{1}{2}\,1$
$^6A_1\,\frac{1}{2}$	$^6A_1\,-\frac{1}{2}$	$-\left(\frac{6}{5}\right)^{\frac{1}{2}}$	$-\left(\frac{3}{5}\right)^{\frac{1}{2}}$	$-\left(\frac{1}{5}\right)^{\frac{1}{2}}$			
$^6A_1\,-\frac{3}{2}$	$^6A_1\,\frac{3}{2}$				$-\left(\frac{4}{5}\right)^{\frac{1}{2}}$		$-\left(\frac{6}{5}\right)^{\frac{1}{2}}$
$^6A_1\,\frac{5}{2}$	$^6A_1\,-\frac{5}{2}$				$-\sqrt{2}$		

6.3.2 Spin Hamiltonian

The matrix elements in Table 6.4 or 6.5 enable us to ascertain the effect upon $^6A_1$ when there is an admixture from $^4T_1$ through spin-orbit coupling.

Assume first that the $^4T_1$ state has a three-fold orbital degeneracy, as it would if the symmetry were truly cubic. Let this zero-order energy be $E(T_1)$ and let the corresponding zero order energy of $^6A_1$ be $E(A_1)$. Further let

$$E(T_1)-E(A_1)=\Delta E. \tag{6.3.12}$$

Since there is no spin-orbit coupling within the $^6A_1$ term, there is no first-order correction to the energy. The second-order corrections to the energy ($E^{(2)}$) may be read directly from Tables 6.4 and 6.5. In terms of ζ, the spin-orbit coupling constant, they are

$$E^{(2)}\left(^6A_1\,\frac{1}{2}\right)=-\left[\frac{6\,\zeta^2}{5\,\Delta E}+\frac{3\,\zeta^2}{5\,\Delta E}+\frac{\zeta^2}{5\,\Delta E}\right]=-\frac{2\,\zeta^2}{\Delta E}=E^{(2)}\left(^6A_1\,-\frac{1}{2}\right),$$

$$E^{(2)}\left(^6A_1\,\frac{3}{2}\right)=-\left[\frac{4\,\zeta^2}{5\,\Delta E}+\frac{6\,\zeta^2}{5\,\Delta E}\right]=-\frac{2\,\zeta^2}{\Delta E}=E^{(2)}\left(^6A_1\,-\frac{3}{2}\right), \tag{6.3.13}$$

$$E^{(2)}\left(^6A_1\,\frac{5}{2}\right)=-\frac{2\,\zeta^2}{\Delta E}=E^{(2)}\left(^6A_1\,-\frac{5}{2}\right).$$

The six components of $^6A_1$ are each shifted in energy by precisely the same amount, and the $^6A_1$ term remains six-fold degenerate. Despite the fact that this conclusion has been reached on the basis of the second order energy corrections, it is nonetheless true to any order. Thus, provided the $^4T_1$ term remains 3-fold spatially degenerate, it will have no effect whatsoever insofar as removal of degeneracies in $^6A_1$ is concerned. Under these circumstances, an electron-spin resonance experiment would disclose $g_x=g_y=g_z=2$, which contradicts the actual observations. We are thus led to suppose that the symmetry at the site of the iron atom is lower than cubic and that the $^4T_1$ term does not have a 3-fold spatial (orbital) degeneracy.

When the symmetry is reduced from cubic to tetragonal (D_4 or C_{4v}), the ${}^4T_1$ term is split into ${}^4A_2$ and ${}^4E$ (Fig. 6.4); Table 5.11 also shows that it is ${}^4T_1 z$ (or ${}^4T_1 0$) that goes over into ${}^4A_2$ while the other two components of ${}^4T_1$ go over into ${}^4E$. If we let

$$\Delta E_0 = E({}^4A_2) - E({}^6A_1),$$
$$\Delta E_1 = E({}^4E) - E({}^6A_1),$$
(6.3.14)

the second-order energy corrections to the components of ${}^6A_1$ are (Table 6.5)

$$E^{(2)}\left({}^6A_1\,\frac{1}{2}\right) = -\frac{\zeta^2}{5}\left[\frac{6}{\Delta E_0} + \frac{4}{\Delta E_1}\right] = E^{(2)}\left({}^6A_1 - \frac{1}{2}\right),$$

$$E^{(2)}\left({}^6A_1\,\frac{3}{2}\right) = -\frac{\zeta^2}{5}\left[\frac{4}{\Delta E_0} + \frac{6}{\Delta E_1}\right] = E^{(2)}\left({}^6A_1 - \frac{3}{2}\right),$$
(6.3.15)

$$E^{(2)}\left({}^6A_1\,\frac{5}{2}\right) = -\frac{2\zeta^2}{\Delta E_1} = E^{(2)}\left({}^6A_1 - \frac{5}{2}\right).$$

It is seen that ${}^6A_1$ is no longer six-fold degenerate but is split into three doublets which have different energies. The states with $+M_S$ and $-M_S$ are still degenerate and, according to Kramers' theorem, there can be no further removal of degeneracies without the use of magnetic fields. It is convenient to define

$$D = \frac{\zeta^2}{5}\left[\frac{1}{\Delta E_0} - \frac{1}{\Delta E_1}\right],$$
(6.3.16)

whence the energy separations among the components of ${}^6A_1$ become

$$E^{(2)}({}^6A_1 \pm \tfrac{3}{2}) - E^{(2)}({}^6A_1 \pm \tfrac{1}{2}) = 2D,$$
$$E^{(2)}({}^6A_1 \pm \tfrac{5}{2}) - E^{(2)}({}^6A_1 \pm \tfrac{1}{2}) = 6D$$
(6.3.17)

as shown in Figs. 6.4 and 6.5 a.

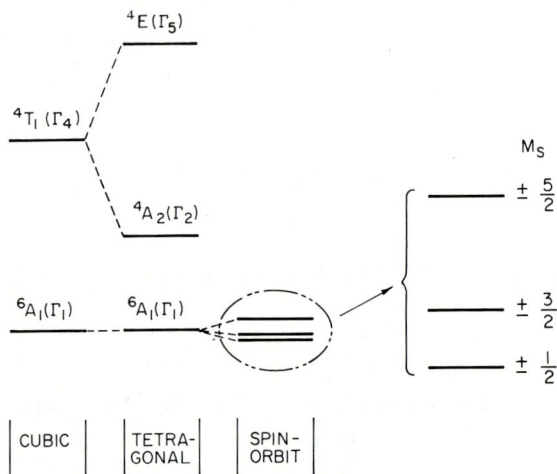

Fig. 6.4. Splitting of ${}^4T_1$ and ${}^6A_1$ under the influence of a tetragonal crystal field and spin-orbit coupling (in second order)

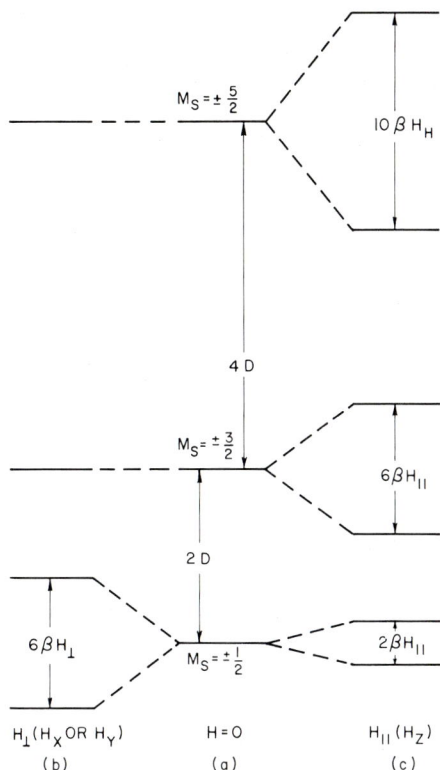

Fig. 6.5 a—c. Splitting of $^6A_1$ in a) zero magnetic field, b) magnetic field perpendicular to the 4-fold axis and c) magnetic field parallel to the 4-fold axis

The level system may also be described by a spin Hamiltonian

$$\mathcal{H}(S) = D(S_z^2 - C),\qquad(6.3.18)$$

in which the constant C is determined by our choice of the zero of energy. For

$$C = \tfrac{1}{3}S(S+1) = \tfrac{35}{12}\quad\text{when}\quad S = \tfrac{5}{2},$$
$$\mathcal{H}(S) = D(S_z^2 - \tfrac{35}{12})\qquad(6.3.19)$$

and the energies of the individual levels are given by

$$E = D(M_S^2 - \tfrac{35}{12})$$

or

$$E = \begin{cases} \tfrac{10}{3}D, & M_S = \pm\tfrac{5}{2}, \\ -\tfrac{2}{3}D & \pm\tfrac{3}{2}, \\ -\tfrac{8}{3}D & \pm\tfrac{1}{2}. \end{cases}\qquad(6.3.20)$$

This puts $E=0$ at the center of gravity of the three levels. Alternatively we can put $C=\tfrac{1}{4}$; then

$$E = \begin{cases} 6D, & M_S = \pm\tfrac{5}{2}, \\ 2D & \pm\tfrac{3}{2}, \\ 0 & \pm\tfrac{1}{2}. \end{cases}\qquad(6.3.21)$$

From (6.3.20) or (6.3.21) it is evident that a convenient labeling for the sub-states of $^6A_1$ is $M_S = \pm\frac{1}{2}, \pm\frac{3}{2}, \pm\frac{5}{2}$.

When the symmetry is reduced still further, as might occur with a rhombic component of the crystal field, the ^4E state is split into two orbitally non-degenerate states, $^4T_1 x$ and $^4T_1 y$. However, the x and y axes would not necessarily be identical with those defined in Fig. 2.1, though they would still in the heme plane if the z axis remained perpendicular to the plane. In that case the spin Hamiltonian, referred to the center of gravity of the $^6A_1$ multiplet, becomes

$$\mathscr{H}(S) = D(S_z^2 - \tfrac{35}{12}) + E(S_x^2 - S_y^2), \tag{6.3.22}$$

where

$$D = \frac{\zeta^2}{4}\left[\frac{1}{\Delta E_0} - \frac{1}{2}\left(\frac{1}{\Delta E_x} + \frac{1}{\Delta E_y}\right)\right], \tag{6.3.23}$$

$$\Delta E_x = E(^4T_1 x) - E(^6A_1),$$
$$\Delta E_y = E(^4T_1 y) - E(^6A_1),$$
$$E = \frac{\zeta^2}{10}\left[\frac{1}{\Delta E_x} - \frac{1}{\Delta E_y}\right]. \tag{6.3.24}$$

The form of D is essentially the same as in (6.3.16) except for the replacement of $1/\Delta E_1$ by the mean value of $1/\Delta E_x$ and $1/\Delta E_y$. The matrix of $\mathscr{H}(S)$ as given in (6.3.22) is shown in Table 6.6.

Table 6.6. *Matrix elements of the spin Hamiltonian $\mathscr{H}(S) = D(S_z^2 - \tfrac{35}{12}) + E(S_x^2 - S_y^2)$ in the basis set $|M_S\rangle = |\pm\frac{1}{2}\rangle, |\pm\frac{3}{2}\rangle$ and $|\pm\frac{5}{2}\rangle$*

		$-\dfrac{1}{2}$	$\dfrac{3}{2}$	$-\dfrac{5}{2}$
		$\dfrac{1}{2}$	$-\dfrac{3}{2}$	$\dfrac{5}{2}$
$-\dfrac{1}{2}$	$\dfrac{1}{2}$	$-\dfrac{8}{3}D$	$3\sqrt{2}E$	$\sqrt{10}E$
$\dfrac{3}{2}$	$-\dfrac{3}{2}$	$3\sqrt{2}E$	$-\dfrac{2}{3}D$	0
$-\dfrac{5}{2}$	$\dfrac{5}{2}$	$\sqrt{10}E$	0	$\dfrac{10}{3}D$

In summary it can be said that if the crystal field is rigorously cubic, both D and E (not to be confused with the energy) are zero and there is no zero-field splitting; however, there may be small contribution from a spin Hamiltonian containing quartic terms. For a tetragonal field $E = 0$; in this case, to second order in spin-orbit coupling, the three levels of $^6A_1$ are pure eigenstates of S_z with $M_S = \pm\frac{1}{2}, \pm\frac{3}{2}, \pm\frac{5}{2}$ and $S = \frac{5}{2}$. Should the ligand field have a rhombic component, D will remain unaffected but E will no longer be zero. The ground term, $^6A_1$, will still consist of three Kramers doublets but they will no longer be pure eigenstates of S_z; since, experimentally, $|E|/D \ll 1$ (Table 6.2), the symmetry is almost tetragonal.

6.3.3 Interaction with a Magnetic Field

To calculate g values it is necessary to compute matrix elements of the magnetic interaction (5.4.7) within the substates of $^6A_1$. Since $L=0$, the interaction Hamiltonian reduces to

$$\mathscr{H}_m = 2\beta\,\mathbf{H}\cdot\mathbf{S} \qquad (6.3.25)$$

or

$$\mathscr{H}_m = 2\beta\,[H_0 S_0 - (H_{+1} S_{-1} + H_{-1} S_{+1})] \qquad (6.3.26)$$

where, in analogy with (5.4.4),

$$S_{\pm 1} = \mp \frac{1}{\sqrt{2}}(S_x \pm i S_y), \qquad S_0 = S_z \qquad (6.3.27)$$

and the components of $\mathbf{H}$ are defined in similar fashion.

We shall set $E=0$ (since $|E|/D \ll 1$) in the spin Hamiltonian (6.3.22); the matrix elements of $\mathscr{H}_m$ are then readily calculated with the aid of the shift operators, as in (5.4.5). The results are given in Table 6.7.

For a magnetic field in the z direction, taken along the 4-fold axis perpendicular to the porphyrin plane, the nonvanishing matrix elements are all on the diagonal. Therefore the energies of the components of $^6A_1$ are

$$E = \begin{cases} \frac{10}{3}D \pm 5\beta H_\parallel, & M_S = \pm\frac{5}{2}, \\ -\frac{2}{3}D \pm 3\beta H_\parallel, & \pm\frac{3}{2}, \\ -\frac{8}{3}D \pm \beta H_\parallel; & \pm\frac{1}{2} \end{cases} \qquad (6.3.28)$$

where $H_z = H_\parallel$. Since each doublet of $^6A_1$ has been split into two levels, all degeneracies have now been removed as shown in Fig. 6.5c. Each level is a pure eigenstate of S_z and there is no mixing of eigenstates by the magnetic field.

Table 6.7. *Matrices of* $2\beta\,\mathbf{H}\cdot\mathbf{S}$. *Single entries refer to the z component of the magnetic field; upper and lower entries refer to x and y components respectively*

$M_S \rightarrow$ ↓	$\frac{1}{2}$	$-\frac{1}{2}$	$\frac{3}{2}$	$-\frac{3}{2}$	$\frac{5}{2}$	$-\frac{5}{2}$
$\frac{1}{2}$	βH_z	$3\beta H_x$ $-i3\beta H_y$	$2\sqrt{2}\beta H_x$ $i2\sqrt{2}\beta H_y$			
$-\frac{1}{2}$	$3\beta H_x$ $i3\beta H_y$	$-\beta H_z$		$2\sqrt{2}\beta H_x$ $-i2\sqrt{2}\beta H_y$		
$\frac{3}{2}$	$2\sqrt{2}\beta H_x$ $-i2\sqrt{2}\beta H_y$		$3\beta H_z$		$\sqrt{5}\beta H_x$ $i\sqrt{5}\beta H_y$	
$-\frac{3}{2}$		$2\sqrt{2}\beta H_x$ $i2\sqrt{2}\beta H_y$		$-3\beta H_z$		$\sqrt{5}\beta H_x$ $-i\sqrt{5}\beta H_y$
$\frac{5}{2}$			$\sqrt{5}\beta H_x$ $-i\sqrt{5}\beta H_y$		$5\beta H_z$	
$-\frac{5}{2}$				$\sqrt{5}\beta H_x$ $i\sqrt{5}\beta H_y$		$-5\beta H_z$

Transitions between magnetic substates are restricted by the selection rules $\Delta M_S = \pm 1$; therefore the only allowed transitions are those between the magnetic substates of the lowest doublet which are separated in energy by $2\beta H_\parallel$. From (6.1.1) we have

$$\hbar\omega = 2\beta H_\parallel = g\beta H_\parallel . \qquad (6.3.29)$$

Hence

$$g_\parallel = g_z = 2 . \qquad (6.3.30)$$

Transitions between the magnetic substates of the doublets with $M_S = \pm\frac{3}{2}$ and $\pm\frac{5}{2}$ are forbidden, though if the magnetic field were high enough in relation to D, transitions between adjacent substates like $|-\frac{3}{2}\rangle$ and $|-\frac{1}{2}\rangle$ could conceivably occur. Since there does not appear to be any experimental evidence for such transitions it can be concluded that D is of the order of a few cm^{-1}.

For a magnetic field in the xy plane ($H_\perp$) the magnetic Hamiltonian (6.3.25) is

$$\mathscr{H}_m = 2\beta H_\perp (S_x \cos\varphi + S_y \sin\varphi) \qquad (6.3.31)$$

where φ is the azimuth angle. In this case we find only off-diagonal matrix elements for $\mathscr{H}_m$ (Table 6.7). To first order, there is no splitting of the doublets $|\pm\frac{3}{2}\rangle$ and $|\pm\frac{5}{2}\rangle$ while the splitting in $|\pm\frac{1}{2}\rangle$ is obtained by diagonalizing

$$\begin{pmatrix} 0 & 3\beta H_\perp e^{i\varphi} \\ 3\beta H_\perp e^{i\varphi} & 0 \end{pmatrix} .$$

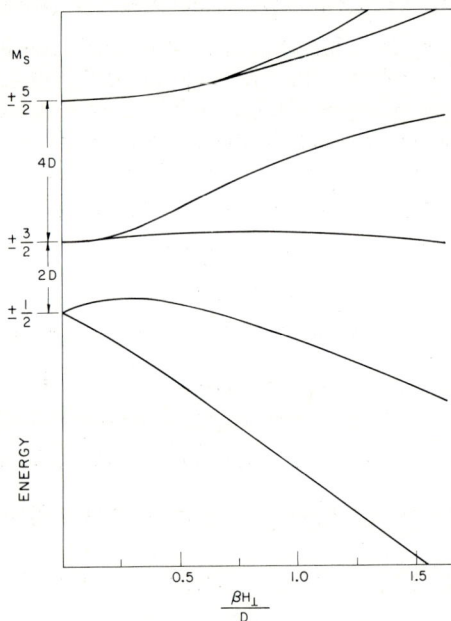

Fig. 6.6. Energies of the magnetic substates of $^6A_1$ as a function of $\beta H_\perp/D$

The difference between the two eigenvalues is $6\beta H_\perp$ which leads, as in (6.3.29), to

$$g_\perp = g_x = g_y = 6 . \tag{6.3.32}$$

To second order, Table 6.7 shows that $H_\perp$ can mix $|\pm\frac{1}{2}\rangle$ with $|\pm\frac{3}{2}\rangle$ and $|\pm\frac{3}{2}\rangle$ with $|\pm\frac{5}{2}\rangle$. The energies are

$$E = \begin{cases} \dfrac{10}{3} D + \dfrac{5}{4}\dfrac{\beta^2 H_\perp^2}{D} , \\[2mm] -\dfrac{2}{3} D + \dfrac{11}{4}\dfrac{\beta^2 H_\perp^2}{D} , \\[2mm] -\dfrac{8}{3} D \pm 3\beta H_\perp - \dfrac{4\beta^2 H_\perp^2}{D} . \end{cases} \tag{6.3.33}$$

As a final step, it is certainly possible to diagonalize, numerically, the 6×6 matrix associated with the application of $H_\perp$; this will then be the solution to all orders in $H_\perp$ and will include (6.3.33) as a special case. The eigenvalues are plotted in Fig. 6.6 as a function of $\beta H_\perp/D$.

6.4 Paramagnetic Susceptibility

ESR experiments in both low- and high-spin ferrihemoglobin have provided us with a knowledge of the level structure in the vicinity of their respective ground states and the behavior of these levels in external magnetic fields. It is therefore possible to derive expressions for the paramagnetic susceptibility or equivalently for the effective Bohr magneton number by means of the defining equation (6.1.7).

6.4.1 Low-Spin Ferrihemoglobin

The energy-level system for this case (Fig. 6.3) consists of three widely-separated Kramers doublets with the uppermost doublet sufficiently elevated in energy for its electronic population to be safely ignored. If we confine our attention to the first and second doublet, the energies in a magnetic field are obtained from (6.2.2) and (6.2.6) to first order in H. They are

$$\begin{aligned} H = H_x, \quad & E_1^x = \pm\beta H_x[(B_1+C_1)^2 - A_1^2], \\ & E_2^x = 2.61\,\lambda \pm \beta H_x[(B_2+C_2)^2 - A_2^2]; \\[2mm] H = H_y, \quad & E_1^y = \pm\beta H_y[(A_1-C_1)^2 - B_1^2], \\ & E_2^y = 2.61\,\lambda \pm \beta H_y[(A_2-C_2)^2 - B_2^2]; \\[2mm] H = H_z, \quad & E_1^z = \pm\beta H_z[(A_1-B_1)^2 - C_1^2], \\ & E_2^z = 2.61\,\lambda \pm \beta H_z[(A_2-B_2)^2 - C_2^2]. \end{aligned} \tag{6.4.1}$$

Numerical values of the coefficients are given in (6.2.18); substitution in (6.1.7) leads to

$$\begin{aligned} H = H_x, \quad & n_e^2 = \frac{3}{1+q}\left[(0.853)^2 + (1.112)^2\, q\right], \\[2mm] H = H_y, \quad & n_e^2 = \frac{3}{1+q}\left[(1.101)^2 + (0.928)^2\, q\right], \\[2mm] H = H_z, \quad & n_e^2 = \frac{3}{1+q}\left[(1.388)^2 + (0.551)^2\, q\right] \end{aligned} \tag{6.4.2}$$

where

$$q = e^{-2.61\,\lambda/kT}\,.$$

As $T \to 0$, $q \to 0$ and the average value of n_e becomes

$$n_e(\text{av}) = \sqrt{3.87} = 1.97 \qquad (T \to 0)\,. \tag{6.4.3}$$

Since most of the population resides in the lowest doublet even at room temperature, the value of n_e obtained above is not far from the room temperature value $n_e(T = 300\,^\circ\text{K}) = 2.13$, which can be compared with the spin-only value of 1.73 for $S = \tfrac{1}{2}$.

The calculation may be carried to second order in H by computing the 6×6 matrix of $l + 2s$ within the set $\psi_{\frac{1}{2}}^{\pm}$, $\psi_{\frac{3}{2}}^{\pm}$ and $\psi_{\frac{5}{2}}^{\pm}$. The basic information is contained in Table 5.16. KOTANI (1961) gives the expressions for n_e^2 when the energies are expressed to second order in H.

6.4.2 High-Spin Ferrihemoglobin

For a magnetic field $(H_{\parallel})$ parallel to the 4-fold axis (z direction), the energies of the low-lying states are given by (6.3.28). According to (6.1.7) and (6.1.11) the effective Bohr magneton number is given by

$$n_e^2(\parallel) = \frac{3(1 + 9e^{-2x} + 25e^{-6x})}{1 + e^{-2x} + e^{-6x}} \tag{6.4.4}$$

with

$$x = \frac{D}{kT}\,.$$

When the temperature is high $(x \to 0)$

$$n_e(\parallel) = \sqrt{35} = 5.92 \qquad (T \to \infty)\,, \tag{6.4.5}$$

which corresponds to the spin-only value (Table 6.1) for $S = 5/2$. In the opposite limit, at low temperatures $(x \to \infty)$

$$n_e(\parallel) = \sqrt{3} = 1.73 \qquad (T \to 0)\,, \tag{6.4.6}$$

which corresponds to the spin-only value $S = 1/2$.

When the magnetic field is in the heme plane $(H_{\perp})$ the energies are given to second order in H by (6.3.33). We then obtain

$$n_e^2(\perp) = \frac{3\left[9 + \dfrac{8}{x} - \dfrac{11}{2x}e^{-2x} - \dfrac{5}{2x}e^{-6x}\right]}{1 + e^{-2x} + e^{-6x}}\,. \tag{6.4.7}$$

In the limits of high and low temperature

$$\begin{aligned} n_e(\perp) = n_e(\parallel) = \sqrt{35} = 5.92 \qquad & (T \to \infty)\,, \\ n_e(\perp) = 3\sqrt{3} = 5.19 \qquad & (T \to 0)\,. \end{aligned} \tag{6.4.8}$$

For polycrystalline samples, n_e^2 is a weighted average of $n_e^2(\|)$ and $n_e^2(\perp)$ with weights of $\frac{1}{3}$ and $\frac{2}{3}$ respectively. This gives

$$n_e^2(\text{av}) = \frac{19 + \dfrac{16}{x} + \left(9 - \dfrac{11}{x}\right)e^{-2x} + \left(25 - \dfrac{5}{x}\right)e^{-6x}}{1 + e^{-2x} + e^{-6x}} \qquad (6.4.9)$$

and

$$n_e(\text{av}) = \sqrt{35} = 5.92 \qquad (T \to \infty),$$

$$n_e(\text{av}) = \sqrt{19} = 4.36 \qquad (T \to 0).$$

KOTANI (1961, 1968) shows plots of (6.4.4), (6.4.7), and (6.4.9).

These results are readily understood from the level diagram Fig. 6.5. In the high temperature limit, the populations in the three doublets tend to equalize so that in spite of their energy separations the three doublets contribute to the susceptibility precisely as would a 6-fold degenerate state with $S = 5/2$; it then makes no difference in what direction the magnetic field is applied. At the low temperature limit, only the lowest doublet with $|M_S\rangle = |\pm\frac{1}{2}\rangle$ is occupied and the others are vacant. When the field is parallel to the z axis the system behaves like a free spin $(g_{\|} = 2)$ with $S = \frac{1}{2}$ while for a perpendicular field the susceptibility also increases by the same factor (to first order in H) since the splitting is three times larger $(g_{\perp} = 6)$.

6.4.3 Ferrohemoglobin

Measurements of magnetic susceptibility confirm that oxyhemoglobin is diamagnetic; deoxyhemoglobin on the other hand, has a Bohr magneton number, n_e, of 5.4 (Table 6.2). The spin-only value of n_e for $S = 2$ is 4.90; it is therefore reasonable to assume that deoxyhemoglobin is a high-spin complex with $S = 2$ in which there is incomplete quenching of orbital angular momentum to account for the increase in the measured value of n_e over the spin-only value. For the ferrihemoglobin derivatives we were able to derive expressions for the susceptibility or the magneton number based on an energy level structure deduced from electron-spin resonance experiments. For ferrohemoglobin there are no such data; however, theoretical considerations provide some guidance (GRIFFITH, 1961; KOTANI, 1964a).

The ground state of high-spin ferrohemoglobin (Fig. 5.6) is $t_2^4 e^2 \, {}^5T_2$. The effect of spin-orbit coupling is to split ${}^5T_2$ into three levels as if we were dealing with an atomic ${}^5P$ term. In the latter case there are three values of J, namely, 3, 2 and 1, and the levels have degeneracies of 7, 5, and 3 respectively. The energies follow the Landé interval rule. Precisely the same thing occurs with ${}^5T_2$. GRIFFITH (1961) computes n_e^2 for this level structure:

$$n_e^2 = \frac{3(49x + 108) + 5(27x - 20)e^{-\frac{1}{2}x} + 56(3x - 4)e^{-\frac{5}{4}x}}{2x(3 + 5e^{-\frac{1}{2}x} + 7e^{-\frac{5}{4}x})},$$

$$x = \frac{\zeta}{kT}. \qquad (6.4.10)$$

In the limit of high temperature, $n_e \to 5.3$; as the temperature is lowered, n_e rises slowly to a peak value of about 5.8 and then eventually falls to the spin-only value. At room temperature, the prediction based on (6.4.10) and the observed value are in satisfactory agreement.

6.5 Discussion

We can now summarize what has been learned from magnetic experiments concerning the electronic states of hemoglobin and what this information implies with regard to structural features and physical mechanisms. By far the most important influence on the symmetry of the environment in which the iron atom is immersed is that exerted by the nearest ligands. Nevertheless, less direct effects such as the conformation of the protein or the state of association of the subunits—whether as isolated chains or as dimers or tetramers—should not be entirely ignored.

In low-spin ferrihemoglobin the five $3d$ electrons are all situated in t_2 orbitals (see, however, GRIFFITH, 1971), which are threefold (spatially) degenerate in a cubic field. However, the symmetry around the iron atom is certainly lower than cubic, and indeed lower than tetragonal. In such a crystal field the threefold degeneracy of the t_2 orbitals is completely removed. A second important effect is that of spin-orbit coupling, which mixes the orbitals and produces a set of three Kramers doublets (Fig. 6.3). The $\zeta(d_{xy})$ orbital has the lowest energy; about $1500\,\mathrm{cm}^{-1}$ above it is the $\eta(d_{zx})$ orbital, and about $1000\,\mathrm{cm}^{-1}$ higher yet is the $\xi(d_{yz})$ orbital. The doublet separations are of comparable energy—a situation which is markedly different from that in high-spin ferrihemoglobin, in which there are also three Kramers doublets but with separations approximately one hundred times smaller (Fig. 6.5).

What is the origin of the low-symmetry crystal field in low-spin ferrihemoglobin? One obvious source of asymmetry is the π bonding to imidazole belonging to the heme-linked (proximal) histidine. The attachment of iron to histidine is shown in Fig. 2.2 where it is seen that the plane of the heme and the plane of the imidazole are perpendicular to one another. The normals to the two planes define two perpendicular axes; a third axis may be taken perpendicular to the first two. We see then that in the plane of the porphyrin, the two axes (x and y) are no longer equivalent, so that $g_x \neq g_y$ as is actually observed. As a further step in the argument let us suppose that the imidazole plane is oriented with its normal parallel to the y axis. The $2p\pi$ orbital on the imidazole nitrogen will then have its maxima along the y axis. By analogy with the discussion in Section 5.4, the largest electrostatic repulsion will occur between an electron in the $2p\pi$ orbital and one in the ξ orbital, whereas the smallest repulsion will be with an electron in the ζ orbital which has no lobes protruding out of the xy plane. In Chapter VII the same argument will be expressed in the language of molecular-orbital theory, where it will be shown that the ξ and η orbitals participate more strongly in the formation of an antibonding molecular orbital.

As the strongest repulsion occurs between imidazole (assumed to lie in the xz plane) and the $\xi(d_{yz})$ orbital, the smallest g value should lie along the x direction which corresponds to the projection of imidazole on the heme plane. Thus g_x should be a minimum and g_y a maximum. According to HELCKÉ et al. (1968), these conclusions are supported by crystallographic data.

A numerical estimate by KOTANI (1964 b) of the asymmetry that can be ascribed to the position of the imidazole ring indicated that the ξ and η orbitals would be separated by about $60 \, \mathrm{cm}^{-1}$. This by itself, of course, is far too small to account for the observed rhombic splitting.

In the case of the azide derivative, crystallographic data indicate that the linear azide ion (N_3^-) is inclined at $21°$ to the porphyrin plane (Fig. 2.5). This is another source of asymmetry whose effect has been estimated by KOTANI (1964 b). Clearly such an explanation is not applicable to the many other low-spin derivatives which also have three distinct g values characteristic of a low-symmetry ligand field.

In molecules or complexes with orbitally degenerate electronic ground states it is possible for distortions to occur as a result of the Jahn-Teller effect (Section 5.7). This is exemplified by numerous crystals containing XY_6 covalent complexes. Hence it is of interest to investigate the likelihood of the Jahn-Teller effect contributing to the reduction in symmetry and the resultant anisotropies observed in low-spin ferrihemoglobin. This was done by KAMIMURA and MIZUHASHI (1968) and by MIZUHASI (1969). We have seen (Table 5.11) that $^2T_2$ in O goes over into $^2E + {}^2B_2$ in D_4 (or C_{4v}). The symmetrized product $[E^2]$ in D_4 (or C_{4v}) reduces to $A_1 + B_1 + B_2$. Hence, according to the discussion in Section 5.7, an electronic system in an E state (tetragonal symmetry) can interact with a nondegenerate vibrational mode of B symmetry. The calculation initially proceeded on the assumption that a static Jahn-Teller distortion of the porphyrin was responsible for the large anisotropy in the heme plane. The coupling constant between the electronic and nuclear motion was determined so as to fit the observed anisotropy. However, the calculation revealed that the reduction in energy due to the Jahn-Teller effect was of the same order of magnitude as the zero-point energy of the associated vibrational mode, the latter having been estimated from infrared spectra. Under such circumstances it is not possible for a static Jahn-Teller distortion to occur, although a dynamic effect may still exist. The final conclusion was that the anisotropy in the heme plane of low spin ferrihemoglobin azide is probably due to the combined action of the dynamical Jahn-Teller and the rhombic crystal field produced by the position of the azide and the imidazole.

Turning now to high-spin ferrihemoglobin, we find that $g_x = g_y \neq g_z$; the crystal field must therefore contain a strong tetragonal component described by one of the symmetry groups D_4 or C_{4v}—the latter being applicable when the atom is displaced from the porphyrin plane. A spin Hamiltonian which provides a satisfactory description of ESR experiments is

$$\mathscr{H}(S) = \beta[g_\parallel H_z S_z + g_\perp(H_x S_x + H_y S_y)] \\ + D[S_z^2 - \tfrac{1}{3} S(S+1)] + E(S_x^2 - S_y^2)$$
(6.5.1)

with $S = 5/2$, $g_\parallel = 2$ and $g_\perp = 6$.

In a polycrystalline sample, the heme planes are randomly oriented relative to an externally applied magnetic field. Since there are many more ways for a magnetic field to lie in or near a plane than in or near a particular direction, it is expected, on a purely statistical basis, that the intensity of absorption will be much higher for $H_\perp(H_x, H_y)$ than for $H_\parallel(H_z)$. This feature is evident in the spectrum illustrated in Fig. 6.2.

In zero magnetic field and when $E=0$, the spin Hamiltonian (6.5.1) leads to a set of Kramers doublets; these are pure eigenstates of S_z with $|M_S\rangle = |\pm\frac{1}{2}\rangle$, $|\pm\frac{3}{2}\rangle$ and $|\pm\frac{5}{2}\rangle$. If $D>0$, the $|\pm\frac{1}{2}\rangle$ doublet has the lowest energy (Fig. 6.5a), whereas for $D<0$ the level system is inverted. Experimentally, it is found that apart from small refinements due to slight mixing among the doublets, the ESR transitions and the corresponding g values are satisfactorily explained on the basis of magnetic dipole transitions between $|+\frac{1}{2}\rangle$ and $|-\frac{1}{2}\rangle$. Since these transitions do not get weaker as the temperature is lowered, it follows that $D>0$. Were the level system inverted ($D<0$), the population in the $|\pm\frac{1}{2}\rangle$ doublet would be depleted as the temperature is lowered and the signal would decay. It is sometimes stated that high-spin ferrihemoglobin has an effective spin, S', equal to 1/2. This is merely another way of saying that the ESR transitions are associated almost entirely with the $|\pm\frac{1}{2}\rangle$ doublet.

Experimental values of D for several high-spin compounds are listed in Table 6.2. These were obtained by BRACKETT et al. (1971), who employed far infrared absorption techniques to measure the transition energy between adjacent doublets. Another method is based on the variation of the paramagnetic susceptibility with temperature (TASAKI et al., 1967); in this case one seeks the value of D that will give the best fit of the theoretical expression (6.4.9) to the experimental curve. These methods, as well others, indicate quite clearly that in high-spin ferric hemoglobin and myoglobin, D lies in the range of 5 —10 cm^{-1}, which means that at temperatures below about 20°K most of the population resides in the $|\pm\frac{1}{2}\rangle$ doublet.

The magnitude of D in hemoglobin is surprisingly large when compared with the much smaller values of D (0.01 to 0.1 cm^{-1}) found in numerous ferric high-spin inorganic compounds. Theoretically, the low values of D in the inorganic compounds seem more natural, since as we have seen, ^6S is insensitive to low-symmetry fields and any interaction which contributes to the doublet splitting is of second order or higher. Why, then, is D so much larger in hemoglobin?

We may obtain some insight into this question by attempting to estimate the numerical value of D. The zero field splitting in $^6A_1$, it is recalled, has its origin in the spin-orbit coupling between $^6A_1$ and $^4T_1$ in combination with a tetragonal crystal field which splits $^4T_1$ into $^4E+{}^4A_1$ (Fig. 6.4). Referring to (6.3.16) and (6.3.14) for the definitions of D and the energy differences ΔE_0 and ΔE_1, we shall first make the reasonable assumption that the cubic splitting parameter Δ is approximately equal to Δ_c, the cross-over value for high and low spin states. From (5.5.4) we have

$$\Delta_c(\text{Fe}^{3+}) = \tfrac{1}{2}(15B + 10C) = 31600 \text{ cm}^{-1} \qquad (6.5.2)$$

in which $B=1015$ cm^{-1} and $C=4800$ cm^{-1} (KOTANI, 1968). In addition, from (5.5.3) and (5.5.1)

$$E(^4T_1) - E(^6A_1) = 10B + 6C - \Delta = 7350 \text{ cm}^{-1} \qquad (\Delta = \Delta_c). \qquad (6.5.3)$$

The next assumption (KOTANI, 1964b) is that the energy separation $E(^4E) - E(^4A_2)$ is equal to δ, the tetragonal splitting as derived from ESR experiments on low-spin ferrihemoglobin (6.2.20). The basis for this assumption is found in the expressions for $^4T_1$ in terms of the one-electron orbitals (5.5.11). In a tetragonal field $^4T_1 x$ and $^4T_1 y$ go over into ^4E while $^4T_1 z$ becomes $^4A_2$; therefore

$$E(^4E) - E(^4A_2) = \varepsilon_{\xi,\eta} - \varepsilon_\zeta = \delta = 2060 \text{ cm}^{-1}.$$

For $D > 0$, $^4A_2$ is lower in energy than ^4E; we then have

$$\Delta E_0 = E(^4A_2) - E(^6A_1) = E(^4T_1) - \tfrac{2}{3}\delta - E(^6A_1) = 5980 \text{ cm}^{-1}, \qquad (6.5.4)$$

$$\Delta E_1 = E(^4E) - E(^6A_1) = E(^4T_1) + \tfrac{1}{3}\delta - E(^6A_1) = 8040 \text{ cm}^{-1}. \qquad (6.5.5)$$

Substituting into (6.3.16), with $\zeta = 435 \text{ cm}^{-1}$, we get $D = 1.6 \text{ cm}^{-1}$ which is smaller than the experimental values (Table 6.2) but nevertheless, of the right order of magnitude. Were we to take the experimental values of D, with the tetragonal splitting $\delta = 2060 \text{ cm}^{-1}$, as before, the excitation energy of $^4A_2$ would then be 2000—3000 cm^{-1} in place of the value in (6.5.4).

We now summarize the effect of an external magnetic field, considering first the approximation in which $E = 0$. When the field is applied parallel to the z axis (perpendicular to the heme plane) all the doublets are split into Zeeman levels (Fig. 6.5c) and each level remains an eigenstate of S_z. The selection rule $\Delta M_S = \pm 1$ permits magnetic dipole transitions to occur between $|+\tfrac{1}{2}\rangle$ and $|-\tfrac{1}{2}\rangle$; this is the origin of the ESR signal at $g = 2$. Transitions among the substates of the higher doublets are forbidden. A magnetic field applied perpendicular to the z axis (parallel to the heme plane) produces more complicated effects. When $\beta H \ll D$, the $|\pm\tfrac{1}{2}\rangle$ doublet is split but the higher ones are not (Fig. 6.5b). The transitions which occur in the lowest doublet are the ones observed at $g = 6$. As the magnetic field is increased, the energies of the Zeeman levels in the ground doublet acquire a quadratic dependence on the field; states for which $\Delta M_S = \pm 1$ begin to mix. When $\beta H \approx D$, all the Zeeman levels are thoroughly mixed, so that M_S is no longer a good quantum number; the upper two doublets are now also split, with the splitting of $|\pm\tfrac{3}{2}\rangle$ greater than that of $|\pm\tfrac{5}{2}\rangle$ (Fig. 6.6). Finally when $\beta H \gg D$, order is again restored since the zero field splitting has now become unimportant and each Zeeman level is again an eigenstate of S_z and $g = 2$. In the latter case the g values thus become isotropic.

When $E \neq 0$, the term $E(S_x^2 - S_y^2)$ in (6.5.1) couples states for which $\Delta M_S = \pm 2$. The eigenfunctions are no longer pure eigenstates of S_z, and this admixture is reflected in a shift of the Kramers doublets so that the separations are no longer precisely $2D$ and $4D$ (Fig. 6.5a) but, instead, are functions of E/D. In the presence of a magnetic field it is necessary to diagonalize the complete Hamiltonian (6.5.1). The most important effect is that the absorption line at $g = 6$ broadens or splits into components, that is, g_x and g_y are no longer exactly equal. The difference in the two g values, Δg, for $|E|/D \ll 1$ is given by

$$\Delta g = 48 \frac{|E|}{D}. \qquad (6.5.6)$$

KOTANI and MORIMOTO (1967) employed this relationship to obtain an experimental value of $|E|/D$ in single crystals of metmyoglobin and ferrimyoglobin fluoride. This was accomplished by measuring the anisotropy in the g value with magnetic field maintained parallel to the heme plane but at various azimuth angles. The values obtained in this way (Table 6.2) indeed verified that $|E|/D \ll 1$. In the case of the fluoride derivatives there is an additional broadening or splitting of the ESR lines which arises from a superhyperfine interaction between the unpaired electrons of the iron atom and the magnetic moment of ^{19}F nucleus which has a spin of 1/2. Effects of this type were noted by MORIMOTO and KOTANI (1966) and by PEISACH et al. (1971).

A theoretical estimate of $|E|$ is possible from (6.3.24) and an assumption that the difference between ΔE_x and ΔE_y is given by the rhombic splitting (6.2.20). Alternatively, experimental values of $|E|$ as shown in Table 6.2 can be used in the calculation of rhombic splitting. The result is that in high-spin ferrihemo-globin the rhombic splitting is only a few tens of cm^{-1}—a value which is con-sistent with KOTANI's (1964 b) estimate of the imidazole contribution. We see, then, that the rhombic splitting in high-spin ferrihemoglobin is only a small fraction of the tetragonal splitting, whereas in the low-spin case the two are of comparable magnitude (1000—2000 cm^{-1}). The numerical estimates of D and E lend support to the hypothesis that for hemoglobin $\Delta \approx \Delta_c$ and that there is probably a common origin to the tetragonal splitting in both low- and high-spin hemoglobin. A large rhombic splitting, however, is uniquely characteristic of the low-spin variety.

Departures from complete tetragonality in high-spin derivatives may also depend on the conformation of the protein or on the state of association of the subunits. Thus, for example, PEISACH et al. (1969) observed that in isolated high-spin ferric α chains, $g_\perp$ has two components, 6.18 and 5.78, whereas in the cor-responding tetramer there is no splitting.

The most convincing experimental evidence for the co-existence of high- and low-spin forms of hemoglobin is supplied by magnetic susceptibility data (Table 6.2). The best example is ferrihemoglobin hydroxide, with a magneton number of 4.7, which falls between the high-spin and low-spin values (Table 6.1). One might suppose that this corresponds to three unpaired electrons with $S = \frac{3}{2}$. Though this hypothesis cannot be eliminated out of hand, intermediate spins in octahedral complexes are not favored on theoretical grounds (GRIFFITH, 1956a). The generally accepted viewpoint, following the work of GEORGE et al. (1964) is that the observed magneton number is the result of a thermal equilibrium between high- and low-spin forms. In Chapter VII it will be shown that this assumption leads to a fruitful connection between magnetic susceptibility and optical spectra.

In low-spin ferrimyoglobin azide the magneton number is 3.3, while the spin-only value for $S = \frac{1}{2}$ is 1.73. An orbital contribution cannot account for such a wide difference. IIZUKA and KOTANI (1968) found that the paramagnetic susceptibility obeys the Curie law at low temperatures up to about $-80°C$, above which there are marked deviations. Their interpretation is that there is a thermal equilibrium between high- and low-spin states in this case too.

Chapter VII

Molecular Orbitals and Optical Spectra

Precise molecular orbital calculations on a system as large as an iron-porphyrin complex have so far been unattainable. The real molecular structure must be simplified and idealized in certain respects, and even then it is necessary to introduce a variety of approximations whose validity is often difficult to assess. Quantitative results should therefore be viewed with considerable caution. Despite such deficiencies, molecular orbital calculations provide us with useful conceptual tools for the interpretation of experimental findings.

The molecular orbital approach, as we have already seen in Section 5.8, is aimed at the construction of a wave function which extends over the whole system. For a metallic complex like iron-porphyrin, this includes the iron atom, the conjugated porphyrin ring and any axial ligands that may be present. Electrons which may be described by such wave functions are therefore not confined to any particular atom; rather, they are delocalized and can roam over the entire system. Calculations which deal specifically with iron-porphyrin structures containing axial ligands were performed by ZERNER, GOUTERMAN and KOBAYASHI (ZGK) (1966); the discussion presented here is based on this work.

7.1 Computational Method

7.1.1 Extended Hückel Method with Self-Consistent Charge (EH-SCC)

In the Extended Hückel method the problem is formulated in terms of an eigenvalue equation,

$$\mathscr{H}_{eff}\, \varphi_i = \varepsilon_i\, \varphi_i ; \qquad (7.1.1)$$

$\mathscr{H}_{eff}$ is an effective Hamiltonian whose detailed form, however, need not be specified. The molecular orbitals φ_i, with energies ε_i, are expressed as linear combinations of atomic orbitals (LCAO),

$$\varphi_i = \sum_p \chi_p C_{pi} , \qquad (7.1.2)$$

where χ_p are atomic orbitals and C_{pi} are coefficients. It is convenient to use the Slater approximation for an atomic orbital

$$\chi(n\,l\,m) = N\,r^{n-l}\,e^{-\zeta r}\,Y_{lm}(\theta,\,\varphi) , \qquad (7.1.3)$$

in which N is a normalizing constant, ζ is an orbital exponent selected empirically, $Y_{lm}(\theta,\,\varphi)$ is a spherical harmonic and n corresponds to the principal quantum number. When the expectation value of the energy in (7.1.1) is minimized, a set of homogeneous equations is obtained whose secular equation is

$$\det |H_{pq} - \varepsilon_i S_{pq}| = 0. \tag{7.1.4}$$

S_{pq} is an overlap integral,

$$S_{pq} = \langle \chi_p | \chi_q \rangle \tag{7.1.5}$$

and H_{pq} is the Hamiltonian integral,

$$H_{pq} = \langle \chi_p | \mathcal{H}_{eff} | \chi_q \rangle. \tag{7.1.6}$$

Solutions to (7.1.4) yield the energy eigenvalues; by substitution in the homogeneous equations, one then obtains the normalized solutions for the coefficients which specify the molecular orbitals according to (7.1.2). However, before this program can be carried out, it is necessary to evaluate the integrals in (7.1.5) and (7.1.6). Since the atomic orbitals are given by (7.1.3), it is possible to evaluate the overlap integrals directly; the Hamiltonian integrals, on the other hand, require some form of semi-empiric approximation.

ZERNER *et al.* (1966) employed the Wolfsberg-Helmholtz approximation:

$$H_{pq} = \tfrac{1}{2}(H_{pp} + H_{qq}) S_{pq}[\kappa + (1 - \kappa)\delta_{pq}]. \tag{7.1.7}$$

κ is an interaction parameter which is chosen empirically; H_{pp} is an atomic orbital ionization potential which depends on whether the atom is neutral or charged. The computation starts from the assumption that the atoms are neutral, and values of H_{pp} are chosen according to a prescription which takes into account experimental ionization potentials. It is then possible to solve the secular determinant (7.1.4) and subsequently to obtain the coefficients in (7.1.2); the latter are subjected to a Mulliken population analysis which establishes the charges on the various atoms. The values of H_{pp} are then readjusted to reflect the fact that the atoms are not neutral and the coefficients are recalculated. When the calculated atomic charges agree with the assumed charges to within a certain accuracy the computation is stopped. This iterative procedure is the essence of the Self-Consistent Charge (SCC) method. The final results provide a set of molecular orbitals—expressed as linear combinations of atomic orbitals—and the corresponding orbital energies. The lowest energy configuration is obtained by distributing all the available electrons among the lowest set of molecular orbitals in accordance with the Pauli principle and taking into account contributions from exchange interactions. However, additional considerations may at times require that some electrons be placed in higher energy orbitals (ZERNER *et al.*, 1966).

7.1.2 Symmetry Considerations

Molecular orbital calculations are best started by organizing the atomic orbitals into linear combinations which transform according to the irreducible representations of the symmetry group. These are the symmetry orbitals mentioned in Section 5.8. The Hamiltonian matrix with the symmetry orbitals as the basis set contains the least number of integrals when compared with the same matrix in another basis set. This is an important computational advantage, particularly when the system is large.

For purposes of illustration, we shall now describe how to construct symmetry orbitals for a simplified iron-porphyrin complex without axial ligands. It will be assumed that the peripheral substituents which distinguish one porphyrin from another have been removed so that the model consists of an iron atom situated in the center of a porphyrin skeleton consisting of 4 nitrogens

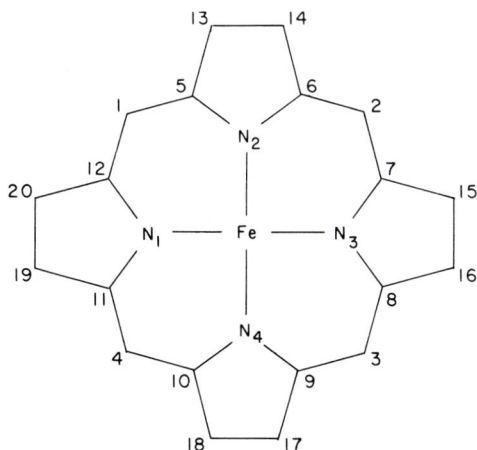

Fig. 7.1. Porphin structure and numbering system

Table 7.1. *Character table for the group D_{4h}*

D_{4h}	E	$2C_4$	C_2	$2C_2'$	$2C_2''$	i	$2S_4$	σ_h	$2\sigma_v$	$2\sigma_d$
A_{1g}	1	1	1	1	1	1	1	1	1	1
A_{2g}	1	1	1	-1	-1	1	1	1	-1	-1
B_{1g}	1	-1	1	1	-1	1	-1	1	1	-1
B_{2g}	1	-1	1	-1	1	1	-1	1	-1	1
E_g	2	0	-2	0	0	2	0	-2	0	0
A_{1u}	1	1	1	1	1	-1	-1	-1	-1	-1
A_{2u}	1	1	1	-1	-1	-1	-1	-1	1	1
B_{1u}	1	-1	1	1	-1	-1	1	-1	-1	1
B_{2u}	1	-1	1	-1	1	-1	1	-1	1	-1
E_u	2	0	-2	0	0	-2	0	2	0	0

Definitions (based on the z axis along the 4-fold symmetry axis)

E: identity operation
C_2: a rotation of 180° about the z axis
C_4: a rotation of ±90° about the z axis
C_2': a rotation of 180° about the x or y axis
C_2'': a rotation of 180° about an axis inclined at 45° to the x and y axis.

σ_h: reflection in the xy plane
i: inversion in the origin ($\sigma_h C_2$)
S_4: combined rotation of ±90° about the z axis with reflection in the xy plane ($\sigma_h C_4$)
σ_v: reflection in the xz or yz plane ($\sigma_h C_2'$)
σ_d: reflection in a plane inclined at 45° to both the xz and yz plane ($\sigma_h C_2''$).

The group D_4 contains the elements E, $2C_4$, C_2, $2C_2'$, $2C_2''$.

Table 7.2. *Symmetry orbitals for the porphin structure shown in Fig. 7.1. The basis set consists of the follow-*

	Fe	$\sigma_{N_1...N_4}$	$\pi_{N_1...N_4}$	$\pi_{C_1...C_4}$
A_{1g}	$4s$ $3d_{z^2}$	$\frac{1}{2}(N_1+N_2+N_3+N_4)$		
A_{2g}				
B_{1g}	$3d_{x^2-y^2}$	$\frac{1}{2}(N_1-N_2+N_3-N_4)$		
B_{2g}	$3d_{xy}$			
E_g	$3d_{yz}$ $3d_{zx}$		$\frac{1}{\sqrt{2}}(N_2-N_4)$ $\frac{1}{\sqrt{2}}(N_1-N_3)$	$\frac{1}{2}(C_1+C_2-C_3-C_4)$ $\frac{1}{2}(C_1-C_2-C_3+C_4)$
A_{1u}				
A_{2u}	$4p_z$		$\frac{1}{2}(N_1+N_2+N_3+N_4)$	$\frac{1}{2}(C_1+C_2+C_3+C_4)$
B_{1u}				$\frac{1}{2}(C_1-C_2+C_3-C_4)$
B_{2u}			$\frac{1}{2}(N_1-N_2+N_3-N_4)$	
E_u	$4p_x$ $4p_y$	$\frac{1}{\sqrt{2}}(N_2-N_4)$ $\frac{1}{\sqrt{2}}(N_1-N_3)$		

ing orbitals: 3d, 4s and 4p on iron, sp² and 2pπ on each of four nitrogens and 2pπ on each of twenty carbons

$\pi_{C_5 \dots C_{12}}$	$\pi_{C_{13} \dots C_{20}}$

$$\left. \begin{array}{l} \frac{1}{2}(C_7 + C_8 - C_{11} - C_{12}) \\[2mm] \frac{1}{2}(C_5 + C_6 - C_9 - C_{10}) \end{array} \right\}$$

$$\left. \begin{array}{l} \frac{1}{2}(C_5 - C_6 - C_9 + C_{10}) \\[2mm] \frac{1}{2}(C_7 - C_8 - C_{11} + C_{12}) \end{array} \right\}$$

$$\frac{1}{2\sqrt{2}}(C_5 - C_6 + C_7 - C_8 + C_9 - C_{10} + C_{11} - C_{12})$$

$$\frac{1}{2\sqrt{2}}(C_5 + C_6 + C_7 + C_8 + C_9 + C_{10} + C_{11} + C_{12})$$

$$\frac{1}{2\sqrt{2}}(C_5 - C_6 - C_7 + C_8 + C_9 - C_{10} - C_{11} + C_{12})$$

$$\frac{1}{2\sqrt{2}}(C_5 + C_6 - C_7 - C_8 + C_9 + C_{10} - C_{11} - C_{12})$$

$$\left. \begin{array}{l} \frac{1}{2}(C_{15} + C_{16} - C_{19} - C_{20}) \\[2mm] \frac{1}{2}(C_{13} + C_{14} - C_{17} - C_{18}) \end{array} \right\}$$

$$\left. \begin{array}{l} \frac{1}{2}(C_{13} - C_{14} - C_{17} + C_{18}) \\[2mm] \frac{1}{2}(C_{15} - C_{16} - C_{19} + C_{20}) \end{array} \right\}$$

$$\frac{1}{2\sqrt{2}}(C_{13} - C_{14} + C_{15} - C_{16} + C_{17} - C_{18} + C_{19} - C_{20})$$

$$\frac{1}{2\sqrt{2}}(C_{13} + C_{14} + C_{15} + C_{16} + C_{17} + C_{18} + C_{19} + C_{20})$$

$$\frac{1}{2\sqrt{2}}(C_{13} - C_{14} - C_{15} + C_{16} + C_{17} - C_{18} - C_{19} + C_{20})$$

$$\frac{1}{2\sqrt{2}}(C_{13} + C_{14} - C_{15} - C_{16} + C_{17} + C_{18} - C_{19} - C_{20})$$

and 20 carbons as shown in Fig. 7.1. The symmetry group is D_{4h}, whose character table is given in Table 7.1.

Both σ and π bonds must be considered. It is assumed that each of the four (in-plane) nitrogen atoms forms a σ bond with iron; the nitrogen orbitals are taken as hybridized sp^2 σ orbitals. For π bonds, it is assumed that each of the four nitrogen atoms contributes a $2p\pi$ orbital and each of the 20 carbon atoms also contributes a $2p\pi$ orbital.

The set of σ orbitals and the set of π orbitals must now be organized into linear combinations which are basis functions for irreducible representations of the group D_{4h}. The four nitrogen σ orbitals constitute a basis set for a reducible representation, $\Gamma(\sigma)$ of the symmetry group D_{4h}; the characters are

D_{4h}	E	$2C_4$	C_2	$2C_2'$	$2C_2''$	i	$2S_4$	σ_h	$2\sigma_v$	$2\sigma_d$
$\chi(\sigma)$	4	0	0	2	0	0	0	4	2	0.

According to (5.2.3) and (5.2.4), the reduction of $\Gamma(\sigma)$ then gives

$$\Gamma(\sigma) = A_{1g} + B_{1g} + E_u.$$

The 24 π orbitals must first be subdivided into sets such that the atoms are equivalent, i.e. connected by a symmetry transformation, within any set. Each set will then be a basis set for a reducible representation of D_{4h}. There are four such sets of equivalent π orbitals: $N_1 \ldots N_4$, $C_1 \ldots C_4$, $C_5 \ldots C_{12}$, and $C_{13} \ldots C_{20}$ where the numbering system is that of Fig. 7.1. The characters of these reducible representations are the following:

D_{4h}	E	$2C_4$	C_2	$2C_2'$	$2C_2''$	i	$2S_4$	σ_h	$2\sigma_v$	$2\sigma_d$
$\chi(\pi_{N_1 \ldots N_4})$	4	0	0	-2	0	0	0	-4	2	0
$\chi(\pi_{C_1 \ldots C_4})$	4	0	0	0	-2	0	0	-4	0	2
$\chi(\pi_{C_5 \ldots C_{12}})$	8	0	0	0	0	0	0	-8	0	0
$\chi(\pi_{C_{13} \ldots C_{20}})$	8	0	0	0	0	0	0	-8	0	0.

The reduction into irreducible representations of D_{4h} gives

$$\Gamma(\pi_{N_1 \ldots N_4}) = A_{2u} + B_{2u} + E_g,$$
$$\Gamma(\pi_{C_1 \ldots C_4}) = A_{2u} + B_{1u} + E_g,$$
$$\Gamma(\pi_{C_5 \ldots C_{12}}) = A_{1u} + A_{2u} + B_{1u} + B_{2u} + 2E_g,$$
$$\Gamma(\pi_{C_{13} \ldots C_{20}}) = A_{1u} + A_{2u} + B_{1u} + B_{2u} + 2E_g,$$

and the linear combinations which belong to each of the irreducible representations are shown in Table 7.2, (OHNO et al., 1963).

When the out-of-plane ligands are added the symmetry is no longer D_{4h}, since operations like C_2' and C_2'' are no longer symmetry elements. In place of D_{4h} the appropriate symmetry group is C_{4v}, which contains the operations $E, 2C_4, C_2, 2\sigma_v$ and $2\sigma_d$ (defined in Table 7.1). We note that these operations are included in D_{4h} so the characters of C_{4v} can be read directly from Table 7.1. For example, the representations A_{1g} and A_{2u} have the same characters for the set of elements in C_{4v}. Therefore A_{1g} and A_{2u} in D_{4h} both correspond to A_1, the totally symmetric representation in C_{4v}. Continuing in this fashion we find that every representation in D_{4h} can be given a label in C_{4v}, or even in C_{2v} if the symmetry is reduced still further. The correspondence between labels is the following:

D_{4h}	C_{4v}	C_{2v}
A_{1g}, A_{2u}	A_1	A_1
A_{2g}, A_{1u}	A_2	A_2
B_{1g}, B_{2u}	B_1	A_1
B_{2g}, B_{1u}	B_2	A_2
E_g, E_u	E	B_1, B_2.

As a consequence, the symmetry orbitals listed in Table 7.2 according to their D_{4h} classification can also be classified according to C_{4v} or C_{2v}.

Having constructed the symmetry orbitals, the next step is to combine them linearly with the $3d$ orbitals of iron according to (7.1.2), subject to the restriction that in any linear combination all the orbitals—symmetry orbitals and iron orbitals—must transform according to the same irreducible representation of the symmetry group. This, then, is the general form of the molecular orbital whose coefficients are to be determined by the method described in Section 7.1.

7.2 Results of Molecular Orbital Calculations

ZERNER et al. (1966) performed an extensive series of calculations on iron porphins with various axial ligands like H_2O, OH, O_2, CN, etc. The porphin structure is identical with that of porphyrin except for the peripheral side chains; in porphyrin these are methyls, vinyls, etc. (Fig. 2.1), whereas in porphin they are all hydrogens. The system therefore consists of one iron, 4 nitrogens, 20 carbons, 12 hydrogens, and the axial ligands. The complex, as a whole, is assumed to be neutral and the basis set consists of all the valence orbitals: ($3d$, $4s$, $4p$) for iron, ($1s$) for hydrogen, and ($2s$, $2p$) for carbon, nitrogen and oxygen.

It is clear from our previous discussion of the molecular orbital method that calculations on a structure as large as the present one are quite involved and require numerous approximations and parameterizations. Our concern will be mainly with the results of such calculations and their bearing on the interpretation of experimental observations on hemoglobin. We have therefore selected five compounds (Table 7.3) from those calculated by ZGK, which are felt to be relevant to corresponding hemoglobin derivatives at least in some features. The energies and occupations of the top filled and lowest empty molecular orbitals are shown in Fig. 7.2; D_{4h} labels are used except for H_2O—Fe—O_2, which also contains some labels according to C_{2v}. Numerical details are given in Tables 7.4, 7.5, and 7.6.

In four of the five compounds listed there is a single axial ligand, while in the remaining case, H_2O—Fe—O_2, there are two axial ligands. In all five cases, the iron atom is displaced from the porphin plane—toward the oxygen molecule in H_2O—Fe—O_2 or toward the single ligand in the others. We shall first consider the 5 coordinated compounds as a group, leaving the oxygen derivative, which has some special characteristics, to be discussed separately.

Table 7.3. *Iron-porphin compounds and their hemoglobin analogs. Coordinates are those of* ZERNER *et al.* (1966)

Compound	Symmetry	Spin	Atom	Coordinates[a]			Analog
				x	y	z	
$Fe^{2+}-H_2O$	C_{2v}	2	Fe	0.0	0.0	0.492	Deoxyhemoglobin
			O	0.0	0.0	2.582	
			H	0.0	±0.800	3.110	
$Fe^{3+}-CN$	C_{4v}	$\frac{1}{2}$	Fe	0.0	0.0	0.455	Ferrihemoglobin cyanide
			C	0.0	0.0	2.295	
			N	0.0	0.0	3.452	
$Fe^{3+}-OH$	C_{4v}	$\frac{5}{2}$	Fe	0.0	0.0	0.455	Ferrihemoglobin hydroxide
			O	0.0	0.0	2.297	
			H	0.0	0.0	3.281	
$Fe^{2+}-CO$	C_{4v}	0	Fe	0.0	0.0	0.492	Carboxyhemoglobin
			C	0.0	0.0	2.332	
			O	0.0	0.0	3.462	
$H_2O-Fe^{2+}-O_2$	C_{2v}	0	Fe	0.0	0.0	0.492	Oxyhemoglobin
			$O(O_2)$	±0.608	0.0	2.01	
			$O(H_2O)$	0.0	0.0	−2.09	
			H	0.0	±0.800	−2.618	

[a] Origin is at the center of the porphin ring; the z axis is prependicular to the porphin plane

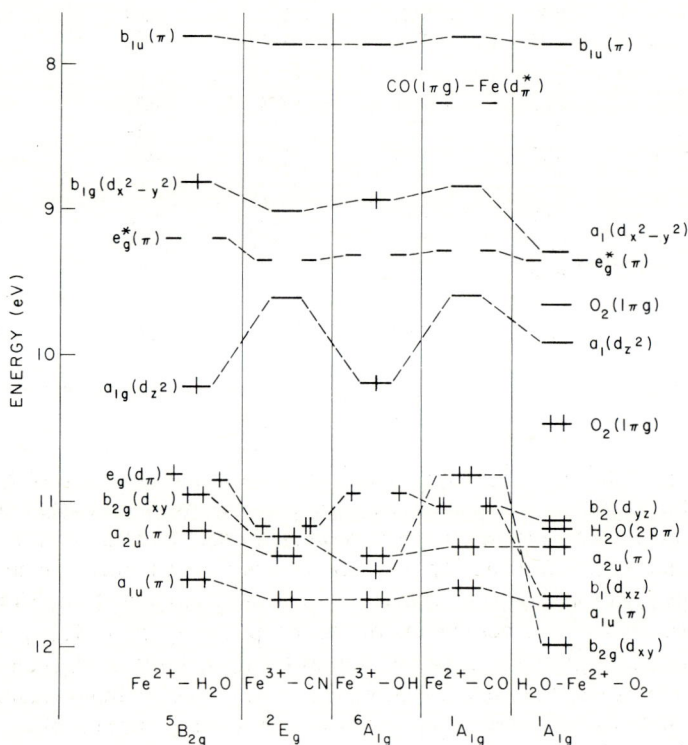

Fig. 7.2. Energies and occupations of molecular orbitals (ZERNER *et al.*, 1966)

Table 7.4. *Atomic composition of iron-porphin molecular orbitals* (ZERNER *et al.*, 1966)

	Fe^{2+}—H_2O	Fe^{3+}—CN	Fe^{3+}—OH	Fe^{2+}—CO	H_2O—Fe^{2+}—O_2
$a_{2u}(\pi)$					
$3d_{z^2}$	0.16	0.07	0.16	0.11	0.02
$4p\pi$	0.03	0.03	0.04	0.02	0.00
Ligands	0.01	0.02	0.02	0.00	0.13
Porphin π	0.79	0.87	0.76	0.86	0.83
$e_{gx}(\pi)$					
$3d_{xz}$	0.01	0.01	0.01	0.01	0.00
Porphin π	0.99	0.99	0.99	0.99	0.99
$e_{gy}(\pi)$					
$3d_{yz}$	0.01	0.01	0.01	0.01	0.01
Porphin π	0.99	0.99	0.99	0.99	0.99
$b_{1g}(d_{x^2-y^2})$					
$3d_{x^2-y^2}$	0.54	0.55	0.46	0.58	
$N(\sigma)$	0.39	0.38	0.46	0.34	
All others	0.07	0.07	0.08	0.08	
$a_{1g}(d_{z^2})$					
$3d_{z^2}$	0.64	0.44	0.55	0.60	0.58
$4s$	0.01	0.00	0.00	0.00	0.00
$4p_z$	0.02	0.13	0.04	0.10	0.02
$N(\sigma)$	0.02	0.04	0.03	0.03	0.07
$N(\pi)$	0.13	0.12	0.17	0.11	0.07
Ligands	0.09	0.20	0.10	0.08	0.18
All others	0.09	0.07	0.11	0.08	0.08
$e_g(d_{xz})$					
$3d_{xz}$	0.83	0.82	0.54	0.76	0.36
Ligands	0.05	0.07	0.33	0.14	0.53
Porphin	0.12	0.11	0.12	0.10	0.10
$e_g(d_{yz})$					
$3d_{yz}$	0.87	0.82	0.54	0.76	0.72
Ligands	0.00	0.07	0.33	0.14	0.11
Porphin	0.13	0.11	0.12	0.10	0.16
$b_{2g}(d_{xy})$					
$3d_{xy}$	0.98	0.98	0.96	0.98	0.79
Porphin	0.02	0.02	0.04	0.02	0.05

Table 7.4 reveals that there are wide differences in the extent to which various atomic orbitals mix with one another in the formation of a molecular orbital. Nevertheless it is seen that there are two broad categories of molecular orbitals: those that are composed mainly of porphin orbitals and those which are predominantly metal orbitals. The notation reflects this classification. Thus, $a_{2u}(\pi)$, $e_{gx}(\pi)$, $e_{gy}(\pi)$ and $a_{1u}(\pi)$ belong mainly to porphin ($a_{1u}(\pi)$ is 100% porphin), while $b_{1g}(d_{x^2y^2})$, $a_{1g}(d_{z^2})$, $e_g(d_\pi)$ (which stands for $e_g(d_{xz})$ and $e_g(d_{yz})$) and $b_{2g}(d_{xy})$ are, to a large extent, the metal $3d$ orbitals. It is this approximate localization of the $3d$ orbitals on the iron atom that accounts for the success of crystal field theory in describing the magnetic properties of metallic complexes.

Whether a complex will be of high or low spin appears to be determined by the position of $a_{1g}(d_{z^2})$. Thus, in both Fe^{3+}—CN and Fe^{2+}—CO the energy of this orbital is considerably higher than in Fe^{3+}—OH and Fe^{2+}—H_2O with the consequence that the former two compounds possess a low spin and the latter a high spin. The ZGK calculations also provide some insight into the structural origin of the spin states. It appears that in a complex with no axial ligands and with the iron in the plane of the porphin the molecular orbital energy

Table 7.5. *Electronic charge distribution in the atomic orbitals of iron* (ZERNER *et al.*, 1966)

	Fe^{2+}—H_2O	Fe^{3+}—CN	Fe^{3+}—OH	Fe^{2+}—CO	H_2O—Fe^{2+}—O_2
$3d_{x^2-y^2}$	1.436	0.881	1.518	0.802	1.004
$3d_{xy}$	1.996	1.995	1.033	1.966	1.996
$3d_{yz}$	1.100	1.496	1.439	1.700	1.982
$3d_{xz}$	1.139	1.496	1.439	1.700	1.240
$3d_{z^2}$	1.331	1.039	1.384	0.725	0.729
Total $3d$	7.002	6.907	6.813	6.923	6.951
$4s$	0.331	0.375	0.356	0.367	0.284
$4p_x$	0.144	0.144	0.166	0.141	0.174
$4p_y$	0.137	0.144	0.166	0.141	0.168
$4p_z$	0.173	0.221	0.249	0.261	0.124
Total $4p$	0.454	0.509	0.581	0.543	0.466
Total Fe	7.787	7.792	7.751	7.832	7.700
Net Fe	0.213	0.208	0.249	0.168	0.300

Table 7.6. *Electronic charge distribution in porphin and ligand orbitals* (ZERNER *et al.*, 1966)

	Fe^{2+}—H_2O	Fe^{3+}—CN	Fe^{3+}—OH	Fe^{2+}—CO	H_2O—Fe^{2+}—O_2
C (2)	4.033	4.005	4.016	4.021	4.020
C (6)	3.984	3.970	3.976	3.976	3.968
C (7)	3.984	3.970	3.976	3.976	3.961
C (14)	4.057	4.047	4.048	4.051	4.046
C (15)	4.057	4.047	4.048	4.051	4.041
N (2)	5.197	5.149	5.193	5.160	5.163
N (3)	5.197	5.149	5.193	5.160	5.142
Total H	11.244	11.212	11.208	11.220	11.192
Total Porphin	112.492	111.961	112.241	112.168	111.951
Net Porphin	−0.492	+0.039	−0.241	−0.168	+0.049
Ligand	H: 0.702 O: 6.322	C: 4.041 N: 5.205	H: 0.709 O: 6.299	C: 3.910 O: 6.091	O(O_2): 6.267 O(H_2O): 6.382 H: 0.716
Net Ligand	+0.274	−0.246	−0.008	−0.001	−0.348

levels are such that d_{xy}, d_{yz}, d_{xy}, and d_{z^2} are close together while $d_{x^2-y^2}$ is of much higher energy. The spin of such a complex has an intermediate value ($S=1$ or $3/2$). When a single axial ligand is added, and the iron atom is kept in the plane of the porphin, d_{z^2} is pushed up to higher energy and the complex acquires a low or intermediate spin. Finally, when the iron is displaced from the porphin plane (with the axial ligand present), $d_{x^2-y^2}$ comes down and the other d orbitals go up; it is then possible for the complex to achieve either high or low—but not intermediate—spin, depending on the nature of the ligand and the magnitude of the displacement. Thus it appears that the displacement of the iron atom from the porphin plane is a necessary condition for a high-spin complex. However, the calculations also show that the energetic balance between high- and low-spin states is very delicate—a characteristic we have already noted.

Another feature of the calculation is that in both ferric and ferrous compounds the charge on the iron atom tends toward neutrality. In the ferric cases the iron atom carries a net positive charge of 0.208 and 0.249 electronic units and in the ferrous, 0.168 and 0.213. It would indeed be difficult to distinguish between ferric and ferrous complexes solely on the basis of the charge on the iron atom.

The compound H_2O—Fe—O_2 differs from the other four listed in Table 7.3 in that it has more than one axial ligand. Two geometries were considered by ZGK:

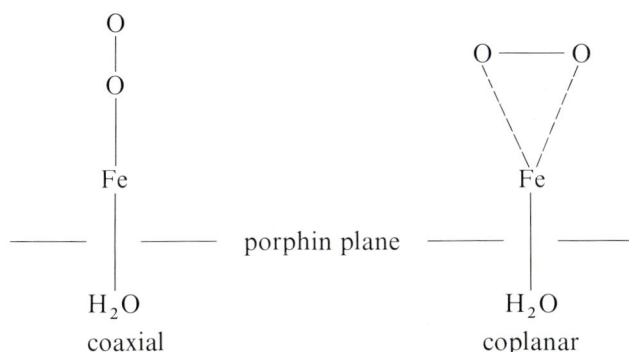

In the coaxial case, the internuclear axis of O_2 is perpendicular to the porphin plane while in the coplanar case the O—O axis lies parallel. In both cases the iron atom is displaced from the porphin plane, in the direction of the oxygen molecule [8].

The coaxial and coplanar structures differ markedly in their properties. It had already been shown by GRIFFITH (1956) that the coaxial structure should be paramagnetic; hence it could not be the structure in oxyhemoglobin which is diamagnetic. The ZGK calculations confirm this conclusion, and moreover suggest that the coaxial form may oxidize to the ferric state and therefore be chemically unstable. On the other hand, the coplanar form is calculated to be diamagnetic and therefore more nearly corresponds to the situation in oxy-

---

[8] This feature of the geometry should be compared with that discussed in Section 2.3.

hemoglobin, though this aspect of the structure remains to be clarified (see Sections 2.3 and 9.1).

The distribution of charge in the coplanar oxygen complex is also noteworthy. The numbers are Fe: 0.30, O_2: -0.534, H_2O: 0.186. The porphin remains essentially neutral; hence it appears that the O_2 ligand accepts electronic charge from both Fe and H_2O, the former being the larger donor. In contrast, the charge on the CO ligand in Fe^{2+}—CO, which is also a ferrous low-spin complex, is only -0.001. The oxygen complex is therefore characterized by the largest migration of charge of any of the complexes calculated by ZGK.

There are also a number of differences in the molecular orbitals. The $3d_{xz}$ metal orbital is thoroughly mixed with orbitals on the axial ligands and, to a lesser extent, with orbitals on the porphin. As a result, $e_g(d_{xz})$ is only 36% metal orbital, which is considerably lower than in the other cases. Also $b_2(d_{xy})$ (or $a_2(d_{xy})$ in C_{2v}) contains only 80% of the metal orbital $3d_{xy}$, again in sharp contrast to the 96—98% for the other complexes.

7.3 Optical Spectra

All proteins absorb strongly in the ultraviolet. At wavelengths of 190—200 nm, the absorption is associated with the peptide bond; at somewhat longer wavelengths—between 260 and 280 nm—the absorption is due to the aromatic group associated with the three amino acids tyrosine, tryptophan, and phenylalanine. Heme proteins have additional absorption bands associated with the

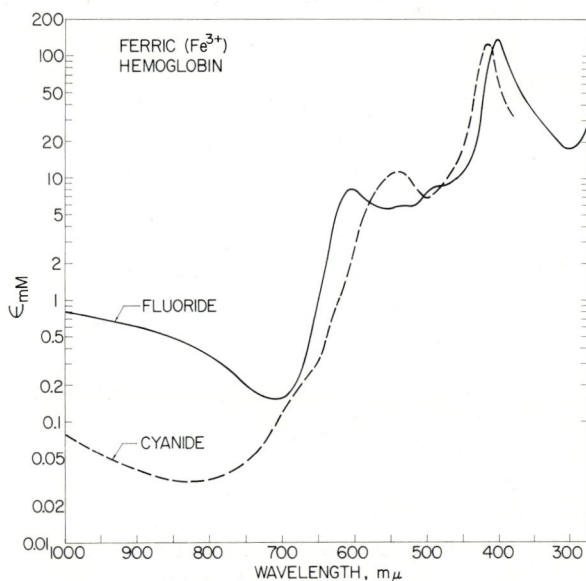

Fig. 7.3. Absorption spectra in ferrihemoglobin fluoride (high-spin) and ferrihemoglobin cyanide (low-spin)

heme group, and it is these which are of primary interest in the spectra of hemoglobin derivatives. Metal porphyrins have spectra which consist of a strong band
in the near ultraviolet (Soret band) and two other bands in the visible; the latter
are responsible for the characteristic red color of most heme proteins. The Soret
band is located at 400—420 nm and has a millimolar extinction coefficient (ε_{mM})
of about 100; the visible bands, generally designated α (longer wavelength) and
β (shorter wavelength), are typically found in the region of 650 and 550 nm
respectively with $\varepsilon_{mM} \sim 10$. These gross features are recognizable in hemoglobin
spectra, though there are significant differences in detail amongst the spectra
of various derivatives. It will therefore be necessary to distinguish between
ferric and ferrous compounds, and even then there will be differences dependent
on the spin and the nature of the axial ligands.

Spectra of ferric and ferrous hemoglobins are shown in Figs. 7.3 and 7.4
respectively, and a summary of the properties of the major bands is given in
Table 7.7. The Soret band is easily recognized as the most intense band with
$\varepsilon_{mM} > 100$. The spectra of oxyhemoglobin and carboxyhemoglobin are very
similar in the visible and near ultraviolet regions; however, in the near infrared,
oxyhemoglobin has a weak, yet distinctive, absorption band centered in the
vicinity of 900 nm, whereas carboxyhemoglobin is essentially transparent in
that region. This is a good example of the high sensitivity of the near infrared
region—in both ferrous and ferric compounds—to a change in axial ligands.
Among the ferric derivatives there are distinct differences in the spectra of high-
and low-spin derivatives. Ferrihemoglobin azide ($S = 1/2$) has a Soret band at
417 nm and α and β bands at 575 and 541 nm respectively. Methemoglobin
($S = 5/2$) has a Soret band at 405 nm and weak α and β bands at 581 and 540 nm
respectively; but, characteristically, there are additional bands at 500, 629 and
1000 nm.

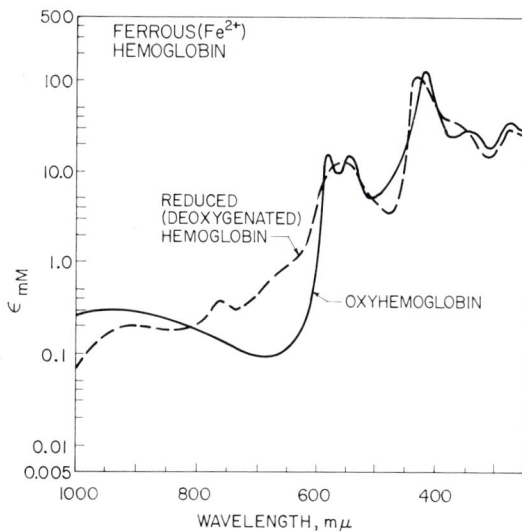

Fig. 7.4. Absorption spectra in deoxyhemoglobin (high-spin) and oxyhemoglobin (low-spin)

Table 7.7. *Some spectroscopic and magnetic properties of hemoglobin derivatives* (ANTONINI *and* BRUNORI, *1970;* SMITH *and* WILLIAMS, *1970*). *The Soret bands are those with* $\varepsilon_{mM} > 100$

	Wavelength nm	Millimolar Extinction Coefficient ε_{mM}	Bohr Magneton Number n_e [a]	Weak Bands nm
Deoxyhemoglobin	555	12.5		590
	430	133		
	274	29.2		
Oxyhemoglobin	541	13.8		920
	577	14.6		
	415	125		
	344	27		
	276	34.4		
Carboxyhemoglobin	540	13.4		
	569	13.4		
	419	191		
	344	28		
Ferrihemoglobin fluoride	840	1.1	5.76	549
	606	10.9		
	490	10.3		
	403	144		
Methemoglobin pH 6.4	1000	0.8	5.65	581
	629	4.4		540
	500	10.0		
	405	179		
Ferrihemoglobin hydroxide	820	0.7	4.66	599
	575	9.2		481
	541	11.0		
	410	120		
Ferrihemoglobin cyanide	541	12.5	2.50	
	418	124		
Ferrihemoglobin azide	575	9.9	2.35	629
	541	12.8		
	417	134		

[a] See also Table 6.2.

The spectrum of ferrihemoglobin hydroxide appears to be neither high-spin nor low-spin but an intermediate between the two. Similarly, the magnetic moment (Table 7.7) has an intermediate value. GEORGE *et al.* (1964) assumed that these properties were correlated and that ferrihemoglobin hydroxide was actually a mixture of high- and low-spin forms in thermal equilibrium. On the basis of these assumptions, the observed values of the magnetic susceptibility, χ, and extinction coefficient, ε, can be expressed by the relations

$$\chi = \chi_h \alpha + \chi_l(1-\alpha), \qquad (7.3.1)$$

$$\varepsilon = \varepsilon_h \alpha + \varepsilon_l(1-\alpha), \qquad (7.3.2)$$

where $\chi_h(\chi_l)$ and $\varepsilon_h(\varepsilon_l)$ are empiric values corresponding to representative high-spin (low-spin) derivatives. α and $(1-\alpha)$ are the fractions of high- and low-spin forms respectively in the thermal mixture. In this fashion, GEORGE et al. (1964) were able to predict extinction coefficients from measurements of magnetic susceptibility and vice versa.

The equilibrium between high- and low-spin states is sentitive to various influences—not only temperature but also pH, change of ligand and change of conformation (SMITH and WILLIAMS, 1970). Nor is it confined to ferrihemoglobin hydroxide; rather, it appears to be a general property of ferric hemoproteins. As a further example, we can cite ferrimyoglobin azide, which also has an intermediate magnetic moment at room temperature but at sufficiently low temperatures goes over entirely into a low-spin form (IIZUKA and YONETANI, 1970). Similarly, for most, if not all, ferric derivatives there is a correlation between spectral and magnetic properties. In the case of ferrihemoglobin hydroxide, this took the form of a correlation between extinction coefficients and magnetic susceptibilities. Yet another type of correlation has been observed in the Soret band (SCHELER et al., 1957): band maxima in low-spin derivatives are located at longer wavelengths than in the high-spin forms. Thus, the Soret band in ferrihemoglobin cyanide ($S=1/2$) is at 418 nm while in ferrihemoglobin fluoride ($S=5/2$) it is located at 403 nm. Finally, it should be remarked that theoretically (Section 2.1) we would expect ferrous derivatives also to be mixtures of high- and low-spin forms in thermal equilibrium, though the experimental results are not as clear-cut as in the ferric types.

Molecular orbital theory of iron porphins, when judiciously coupled with experimental information, provides a basis for the interpretation of hemoglobin spectra (ZERNER et al., 1966; SMITH and WILLIAMS, 1970), though too literal an interpretation must not be expected. Molecular orbitals of the iron porphins, as we have already seen, quite often contain large components of either metal orbitals or porphin orbitals. It is therefore convenient to regard the observed spectra as arising from some combination of three possible types of transitions: $d-d$, $\pi-\pi^*$, and charge transfer. A $d-d$ transition is one in which an electron is excited from one molecular orbital to another, both of which are predominantly $3d$ metal orbitals. Strictly speaking, electric dipole transitions between d orbitals are forbidden in D_{4h} symmetry by the parity selection rule because the dipole moment operator is odd and both initial and final states are even. However, magnetic dipole or electric quadrupole transitions are not forbidden. Also, departures from D_{4h} symmetry—C_{4v} or C_{2v}—which may be introduced, for example, by the axial ligands or by the displacement of the iron atom from the porphin plane, have the effect of removing the center of symmetry so that parity is no longer a good quantum number. In such cases, transitions between d orbitals may occur, but the intensity is generally lower than in allowed transitions. $d-d$ bands in high-spin ferric compounds, for example, are observable but extremely weak. $\pi-\pi^*$ transitions, which turn out to be the most important type in hemoglobin spectra, are those which occur between molecular orbitals largely localized on the porphyrin. Finally, we may have transitions involving a molecular orbital mainly localized on the porphyrin and another localized on the metal; this is a charge transfer transition, porphyrin$\rightleftharpoons$metal. More generally, the axial ligands may also be involved in charge transfer transitions.

In hemoglobin, the absorption spectra spanning the visible and near ultra-violet region are due primarily to the allowed $\pi - \pi^*$ transitions (ZERNER et al., 1966)

$$a_{2u}(\pi) \rightarrow e_g^*(\pi),$$
$$a_{1u}(\pi) \rightarrow e_g^*(\pi). \tag{7.3.3}$$

In the ground state of a complex like Fe^{2+}—CO, both $a_{1u}(\pi)$ and $a_{2u}(\pi)$ are doubly occupied while $e_g(\pi)$ is vacant; hence the ground term is $^1A_{1g}$ (Fig. 7.2). The excited state corresponding to the electron configuration $(a_{2u})^1(e_g)^1$ or $(a_{1u})^1(e_g)^1$ has the symmetry E_u, as can easily be verified from Table (7.1). Hence the singlet-singlet transition is described by $^1A_{1g} - {}^1E_u$ and the matrix elements for dipole transitions which govern the intensity of the absorption bands are

$$\langle {}^1A_{1g}|e\,r|{}^1E_u\rangle.$$

The selection rules are now obtained from the transformation properties of r in D_{4h}. Thus, when $r=z$, Table 7.1 may be used to show that z belongs to the representation A_{2u}. Since the product representation $A_{1g} \times A_{2u} \times E_u$ does not contain the totally symmetric representation A_{1g}, the matrix element necessarily vanishes and the transition is therefore symmetry-forbidden. On the other hand, when $r=x$ or y we find that (x, y) belong to E_u and $A_{1g} \times E_u \times E_u$ contains A_{1g}. It is concluded, therefore, that light polarized parallel to the porphyrin plane may be absorbed whereas light polarized perpendicular to the plane may not.

The energy differences associated with the two transitions in (7.3.3) are close to one another. Because of this near-degeneracy it is necessary to take account of configuration interaction. This means that a particular band cannot be attributed to a transition in which a single electron is excited from one molecular orbital to another. Rather, it is necessary to construct a two-fold degenerate state with the form

$$\psi_i = a_i E_u' + b_i E_u'', \tag{7.3.4}$$

where E_u' and E_u'' are molecular states, both having symmetry E_u and arising from the two electronic configurations $(a_{2u})^1(e_g)^1$ and $(a_{1u})^1(e_g)^1$ respectively; a_i and b_i are constants. The matrix element of the Hamiltonian taken between the two configurations provides a measure of the strength of the interaction.

In this way we achieve a new pair of mixed states separated in energy by an amount which depends on the interconfiguration matrix element; each member is twofold degenerate. The state of higher energy is usually designated B and that of lower energy Q. A further important consequence of invoking configuration interaction is that the transition matrix elements $\langle A_{1g}|e\,r|B\rangle$ and $\langle A_{1g}|e\,r|Q\rangle$ are quite different; the one to the higher state (B) is much larger than that to the lower state (Q). On the one-electron model without configuration mixing, the transition matrix elements to each of the two excited states are the same.

The general interpretation of hemoglobin spectra is now the following: the two excited configurations associated with the transitions (7.3.3) each produce excited states with E_u symmetry and of nearly the same energy. Configurational mixing causes the two excited states to separate into one of higher energy, B, and another of lower energy, Q. The transition from the ground state to B is the more intense of the two and is responsible for the Soret band. The longer wavelength region of the spectrum is associated with the lower energy and lower intensity transition from the ground state to Q. Further splitting into $(0-0)$ and $(0-1)$ vibrational bands gives rise to the $\alpha-\beta$ system. This accounts for the gross features of hemoglobin spectra; at a finer level of detail it is necessary to invoke other types of transitions. Thus, while the Soret band is essentially a pure $\pi-\pi^*$ transition, the visible region has some charge transfer character. This comes about as a result of a transition from porphyrin $a_{1u}(\pi)$ and $a_{2u}(\pi)$ to metal $3d_{xz}$ and $3d_{yz}$ which also produce excited states with E_u symmetry. The near infrared bands are mainly the result of charge transfer transitions. In oxyhemoglobin, particularly, the infrared band is due to a charge transfer transition between metal orbitals and orbitals associated with the oxygen molecule.

Chapter VIII

Mossbauer Spectroscopy

8.1 General Features

The presence of the stable isotope ^{57}Fe to an abundance of 2.2% in all natural compounds of iron makes it possible to study hemoglobin by the methods of Mossbauer spectroscopy (WERTHEIM, 1964; GREENWOOD and GIBB, 1971). In such experiments a sample of hemoglobin is exposed to a beam of highly mono-chromatic γ rays emanating from a radioactive source which contains ^{57}Fe nuclei in an excited state (as a daughter product of ^{57}Co). When the radioactive ^{57}Co is embedded in any one of a number of solid matrices, the γ ray line is so narrow that its energy can easily be shifted several linewidths by means of the Doppler effect, that is, by oscillation of the source (or absorber) at moderate velocities. The velocity drive which provides a Doppler shift to the γ ray photons is therefore the analog of the dispersive device such as a prism or grating in optical spectroscopy. At certain velocities corresponding to shifted γ ray energies the absorption of γ photons in ^{57}Fe nuclei (contained in hemoglobin) is ac-companied by transitions from the nuclear ground state to the first excited state. A plot of the transmitted γ ray intensity as a function of Doppler velocity constitutes a Mossbauer spectrum in which characteristic absorptions are ob-served as a decrease in transmitted intensity at certain velocities. The convention is to consider the velocity as positive when the source and absorber are in relative motion toward each other.

The nucleus is sensitive to its surroundings by virtue of being bound to other nuclei and by the presence of various electric and magnetic hyperfine interactions which manifest themselves in certain distinctive features of the absorption spectra. For this reason, Mossbauer spectra vary from one iron compound to another, or for the same compound under various conditions of temperature, aggregation, external magnetic fields, etc. Since hyperfine interactions often reflect certain features of chemical binding, it has been possible to extract useful information on iron-ligand interactions from a study of Mossbauer spectra. In particular, such experiments yield a measure of s-electron density, electric-field gradient, and effective magnetic field at the position of the nucleus in which resonant γ ray absorption occurs.

To obtain ^{57}Fe in the proper excited state, it is necessary to use the radio-active isotope ^{57}Co which decays, with a half-life of 269 days, to the 136 keV excited state of ^{57}Fe. The latter nucleus, in reverting to its own ground state emits three γ rays, one of which has an energy of 14.4 keV; it is this γ ray which is employed in Mossbauer spectroscopy of iron compounds. The essential feature of the Mossbauer effect is that under suitable conditions, as, for example, in a solid, a certain fraction (f) of the emitted (or absorbed) γ rays have a linewidth close to the natural linewidth. The effect depends first of all on the fact that the recoil energy of ^{57}Fe in the course of emitting (or absorbing) a 14.4 keV photon is 2×10^{-3} eV (Table 8.1), whereas the binding energy is of the order of a few eV. Hence the recoil energy is insufficient to eject the ^{57}Fe nucleus from the lattice. Secondly, there exists a non-vanishing probability that the number of lattice phonons will not be altered when the nucleus emits (or absorbs) a photon. The recoil momentum of the photon may therefore be transferred to the entire crystal; this reduces the recoil energy by a factor of N, where N is the number of atoms in the crystal ($\approx 10^{20}$). The γ ray linewidth can then be very close (within a factor of 2) of the width of the excited level which is 4.6×10^{-9} eV, and as a consequence, hyperfine interactions as small as 10^{-8} eV become accessible to observation by Mossbauer techniques. The ^{57}Fe nucleus thus acts as a sensitive, internal probe of the local environment established by various groups of electrons.

Table 8.1. *Mossbauer parameters of* ^{57}*Fe*

Energy of γ-ray transition	14.4 keV
Mean life of excited state (τ)	1.41×10^{-7} sec
Linewidth ($\Gamma = \hbar/\tau$)	4.6×10^{-9} eV $= 0.096$ mm/sec
Multipolarity	Ml
Recoil energy of ^{57}Fe	2×10^{-3} eV
Natural abundance of ^{57}Fe	2.2%
Spin (I) and parity	
ground state	$\frac{1}{2}^-$
excited state	$\frac{3}{2}^-$
g factor (g_n)	
ground state	0.180
excited state	-0.103
Nuclear Bohr magneton (β_n)	5.05×10^{-24} erg/G $= 3.15 \times 10^{-12}$ eV/G
Gyromagnetic ratio $\left(\dfrac{\gamma}{2\pi} = \dfrac{g_n \beta_n}{h} \right)$	
ground state	138 Hz/G
excited state	$-\ 80$ Hz/G
$\delta R/R$	$-(1.4 - 1.8) \times 10^{-3}$
Energy equivalent of Doppler shift	1 mm/sec $= 4.80 \times 10^{-8}$ eV $= 11.61$ MHz
Quadrupole moment (Q)	
ground state	0
excited state	$\sim 0.2 \times 10^{-24}$ cm^2

The quantity f, known as the Debye-Waller (or Lamb-Mossbauer) factor, depends on certain properties of the solid as well as the energy and mean life of the nuclear excited state. The solid need not be crystalline; Mossbauer effects are readily observed in frozen solutions, lyophilized powders, amorphous materials, and even in liquids of high viscosity. It can be shown (FRAUENFELDER, 1962) that

$$f = \exp\left(-\frac{4\pi^2 \langle r^2 \rangle}{\lambda^2} \right) \qquad (8.1.1)$$

where $\langle r^2 \rangle$ is the square of the displacement of the emitting or absorbing atom from its equilibrium position along the direction of the γ ray momentum, averaged over the lifetime of the nuclear excited state; λ is the wavelength of radiation. It can be seen from (8.1.1) that f is large when the scattering center is confined to a region small with respect to the wavelength of the radiation involved. $\langle r^2 \rangle$ decreases with increasing lattice-binding energy; it also decreases as the temperature is lowered. In addition, f is a function of the angle of emission (or incidence) of the γ ray with respect to crystalline or molecular axes if the binding is anisotropic. Hence the intensity of Mossbauer absorption in a single crystal may vary with the orientation of the crystal relative to the direction of the γ ray beam. However, in most cases of biological interest, the samples consist of a large number of microcrystals with no preferred orientation. The value of f for ^{57}Fe in metallic iron is 0.7 at room temperature and increases to about 0.8 at very low temperatures.

The interpretation of Mossbauer spectra is generally based on three types of interactions—isomer shift, quadrupole splitting and magnetic hyperfine interaction. We shall give a brief summary of each one.

8.1.1 Isomer Shift

Experimentally, the isomer shift (also known as the chemical isomer shift), δ, is defined as the position of the center of the Mossbauer absorption spectrum with respect to zero velocity. The measured value of the isomer shift depends on the material in which the radioactive source is embedded; however, the relative shift for two materials whose spectra are obtained with the same source is independent of the matrix material.

The isomer shift arises from the electrostatic (electric monopole) interaction of s electrons with a nucleus of finite dimensions. If E_g is the energy of the nuclear ground state in the approximation that the nucleus is a point charge, then the true ground state energy of a spherical nucleus with radius R_g and a uniform charge distribution is

$$E'_g = E_g + k R_g^2 e |\psi(0)|^2, \tag{8.1.2}$$

where $e|\psi(0)|^2$ is the total electronic charge density within the nuclear volume and k is a proportionality constant. Since nuclear charge distributions generally vary from one nuclear state to another, the energy E'_e of a nuclear excited state of radius R_e is

$$E'_e = E_e + k R_e^2 e |\psi(0)|^2. \tag{8.1.3}$$

The energy of the emitted γ ray will then be

$$E_\gamma = E_0 + k e |\psi(0)|_S^2 (R_e^2 - R_g^2), \tag{8.1.4}$$

where $E_0 = E_e - E_g$ and $|\psi(0)|_S^2$ refers to the electronic charge density at the nucleus when the latter is embedded in the source material. Correspondingly, in the absorber material we have $|\psi(0)|_A^2$, which is generally different from $|\psi(0)|_S^2$. The nuclear properties are independent of the material; hence the transition energy in the absorber, by analogy with (8.1.4), becomes

$$E'_\gamma = E_0 + ke\,|\psi(0)|^2_A(R_e^2 - R_g^2).$$

(8.1.5)

The difference between E_γ and E'_γ is the isomer shift,

$$\delta = ke\,[R_e^2 - R_g^2]\,[|\psi(0)|^2_A - |\psi(0)|^2_S] = K\left(\frac{\delta R}{R}\right)[|\psi(0)|^2_A - |\psi(0)|^2_S]$$

(8.1.6)

where $\delta R = R_e - R_g$, and R is an average nuclear radius. For ^{57}Fe, K is positive and $\delta R/R$ is negative (Table 8.1).

From (8.1.6) it is seen that the isomer shift is a measure of the difference in electronic charge density over the nuclear volume of absorber nuclei as compared with source nuclei. Since s electrons alone have a nonvanishing probability amplitude at the nucleus, it is expected that for $(3d)^n$ configurations

$$|\psi(0)|^2 = \sum_{k=1}^{3} 2|\psi_{ks}(0)|^2.$$

(8.1.7)

According to this relation the isomer shift for all $(3d)^n$ configurations is predicted to be a constant. Experiments, however, indicate that this is not so. There are considerable variations among compounds with different $(3d)^n$ configurations, as well as among different compounds with the same $(3d)^n$ configuration.

The reason for the first type of variation can be understood on the basis of a partial penetration of $3d$ orbitals into core orbitals. Their presence there has the effect of partially shielding the nucleus and thereby modifying the core orbitals. In particular, s orbitals expand slightly, resulting in a reduction of $|\psi(0)|^2$. Therefore an increase in the number of $3d$ electrons decreases $|\psi(0)|^2_A$; from (8.1.6), with $\delta R/R$ negative, the net effect is to increase δ. We should therefore expect ferrous compounds to have larger isomer shifts than ferric and, indeed, this is what is generally observed. The second type of variation in isomer shift, namely that within a single $(3d)^n$ configuration, is interpreted as a covalency effect. By this it is meant that in the iron-ligand complex, for example, a ligand electron partially resides in the $4s$ orbital of iron. This would be the case if there is a molecular orbital composed of ligand orbitals and the iron $4s$ orbital. In that event

$$|\psi(0)|^2 = \sum_{k=1}^{3} |\psi(0)|^2 + x|\psi_{4s}(0)|^2,$$

(8.1.8)

where x is the fraction of $4s$ electron contributed by the ligand to the iron. We see, then, that isomer shifts have a strong dependence on the details of the electronic configuration and, in compounds, on the extent to which electrons are delocalized.

8.1.2 Quadrupole Splitting

The Hamiltonian which describes the interaction between a nuclearquadrupole moment and an electric field gradient is given by

$$\mathcal{H}_Q = \frac{e^2 qQ}{4I(2I-1)}[3I_z^2 - I(I+1) + \eta(I_x^2 - I_y^2)]$$

(8.1.9)

where I_x, I_y and I_z are components of the nuclear spin operator; Q is the nuclear quadrupole moment defined by

$$Q = \langle II| \sum_{p=1}^{Z} (3z_p^2 - r_p^2)|II\rangle. \qquad (8.1.10)$$

The sum is taken over the Z protons in the nucleus and the matrix element is evaluated for a nuclear state described by a spin-quantum number I and projection-quantum number $m_I = I$; Q is positive for a cigar-shaped distribution and negative for one in the shape of a doorknob. The quantity eq is defined by

$$eq = \langle V_{zz}\rangle = \left\langle \left(\frac{\partial^2 V}{\partial z^2}\right)_0 \right\rangle, \qquad (8.1.11)$$

where e is the proton charge, V is the electrostatic potential and the second derivative is evaluated at the nucleus; the expectation value is calculated with respect to electronic wave functions. The coordinate system, with origin at the nucleus, is chosen to coincide with the principal axis system of the traceless symmetric electric field gradient (EFG) tensor

$$E_{ij} = -V_{ij} = -\left(\frac{\partial^2 V}{\partial x_i \partial x_j}\right)_0. \qquad (8.1.12)$$

It is assumed that the principal components are subject to the Laplace equation,

$$V_{xx} + V_{yy} + V_{zz} = 0,$$

and that

$$|V_{zz}| \geqslant |V_{yy}| \geqslant |V_{xx}|.$$

η is an asymmetry parameter defined by

$$eq\eta = \langle V_{xx} - V_{yy}\rangle. \qquad (8.1.13)$$

When the symmetry is either spherical or cubic, $V_{xx} = V_{yy} = V_{zz} = 0$, and the quadrupole interaction vanishes. When there is axial symmetry, the z axis can be chosen to coincide with the principal axis; in this case $V_{xx} = V_{yy}$ and $\eta = 0$. A single parameter, V_{zz}, then suffices to describe the interaction. For systems of lower symmetry it is necessary to use the general expression (8.1.9).

In ^{57}Fe the nuclear ground state has a spin of $\frac{1}{2}$. The matrix elements of $\mathcal{H}_Q$ within the set $|\frac{1}{2}\rangle$, $|-\frac{1}{2}\rangle$ are all zero; hence there is no quadrupole interaction in the ground state. In the first excited state $I = \frac{3}{2}$; the matrix of $\mathcal{H}_Q$ within the manifold of states belonging to $I = \frac{3}{2}$ is shown in Table 8.2. We note that there is only one 2×2 matrix with eigenvalues

$$E_{\pm} = \pm \frac{e^2 qQ}{4}\left(1 + \frac{\eta^2}{3}\right)^{\frac{1}{2}}. \qquad (8.1.14)$$

When $\eta = 0$ the eigenvalues are $|\pm\frac{3}{2}\rangle$ and $|\pm\frac{1}{2}\rangle$ with energies E_+ and E_- respectively—a manifestation of the fact that the energy of a nonspherical charge distribution (nucleus) with $Q \neq 0$ depends on its orientation relative to the components of the electric field gradient. For $\eta \neq 0$, $|+\frac{3}{2}\rangle$ mixes with $|-\frac{1}{2}\rangle$ and

Table 8.2. *Matrix elements (in units of $\frac{1}{4}e^2 qQ$) of the quadrupole interaction Hamiltonian (8.1.9) for $I=\frac{3}{2}$*

$\mathcal{H}_Q$	$\dfrac{3}{2}$	$-\dfrac{1}{2}$	$-\dfrac{3}{2}$	$\dfrac{1}{2}$
$\dfrac{3}{2}$	1	$\dfrac{\eta}{\sqrt{3}}$		
$-\dfrac{1}{2}$	$\dfrac{\eta}{\sqrt{3}}$	-1		
$-\dfrac{3}{2}$			1	$\dfrac{\eta}{\sqrt{3}}$
$\dfrac{1}{2}$			$\dfrac{\eta}{\sqrt{3}}$	-1

$|-\frac{3}{2}\rangle$ with $|+\frac{1}{2}\rangle$. In either case, the 4-fold degenerate state with $I=\frac{3}{2}$ is split by the quadrupole interaction into two 2-fold degenerate states which we label $|\pm\frac{3}{2}\rangle$ and $|\pm\frac{1}{2}\rangle$ even when $\eta\neq0$; the energy separation is

$$\Delta E = \frac{e^2 qQ}{2}\left(1+\frac{\eta^2}{3}\right)^{\frac{1}{2}}. \tag{8.1.15}$$

Transitions from the ground state ($I=\frac{1}{2}$) to each of the two levels belonging to $I=\frac{3}{2}$ produce a spectrum consisting of two lines with separation Δ. Such a doublet is characteristic of the interaction between the quadrupole moment of the excited state of ^{57}Fe and the gradient of the electric field at the nucleus established by surrounding electrons.

The quantity $e^2 qQ$ is known as the quadrupole coupling constant. It can be positive or negative. Since Q is zero in the ground state and positive in the excited state of ^{57}Fe (Table 8.1) we have the following scheme:

$$
\begin{array}{lcc}
e^2 qQ & + & - \\
q & + & - \\
V_{zz} & + & - \\
E(\pm\frac{3}{2})-E(\pm\frac{1}{2}) & + & - .
\end{array}
$$

A measurement of the quadrupole splitting alone does not reveal the sign of the coupling constant; however the sign can often be deduced from other experiments as, for example, the effect on the Mossbauer spectrum of an external magnetic field.

For an electron at x, y, z and a nucleus at the origin, V_{zz} at the nucleus is

$$V_{zz} = \frac{\partial^2}{\partial z^2}\left(-\frac{e}{r}\right) = -e\frac{3z^2-r^2}{r^5} = -e\frac{3\cos^2\theta-1}{r^3}. \tag{8.1.16}$$

When the electron is distributed over an orbital, the expectation value

$$q = \left\langle \frac{V_{zz}}{e} \right\rangle = -\langle 3\cos^2\theta - 1\rangle \left\langle \frac{1}{r^3} \right\rangle \qquad (8.1.17)$$

is the important parameter. One way to perform this computation is to recognize that

$$3\cos^2\theta - 1 = 2\left(\frac{4\pi}{5}\right)^{\frac{1}{2}} Y_{20} \qquad (8.1.18)$$

so that the theorem stated in (5.2.18) can be employed. Similarly,

$$q\eta = \left\langle \frac{V_{zz} - V_{yy}}{e} \right\rangle = -\langle 3\sin^2\theta \cos 2\varphi \rangle \left\langle \frac{1}{r^3} \right\rangle \qquad (8.1.19)$$

with

$$\sin^2\theta \cos 2\varphi = \left(\frac{8\pi}{15}\right)^{\frac{1}{2}} (Y_{22} + Y_{2-2}). \qquad (8.1.20)$$

The numerical values of q and η for p and d orbitals are given in Table 8.3.

Table 8.3. *Electric field gradient parameters of p and d electrons*

Orbital	$q_p/\langle r^{-3}\rangle_p$	η_p
p_x	$\frac{2}{5}$	-3
p_y	$\frac{2}{5}$	3
p_z	$-\frac{4}{5}$	0

	$q_d/\langle r^{-3}\rangle_d$	η_d
$d_{x^2-y^2}$	$\frac{4}{7}$	0
d_{z^2}	$-\frac{4}{7}$	0
d_{xy}	$\frac{4}{7}$	0
d_{zx}	$-\frac{2}{7}$	3
d_{yz}	$-\frac{2}{7}$	-3

It has already been shown on general grounds that both q and η vanish in a cubic field. This may also be verified directly from the form of the cubic potential V_c, as given in (5.2.21), by evaluating the second derivatives at the origin. We may also view this result from the standpoint of the degeneracies in a cubic field. An electron occupying a t_2 orbital has an equal probability of residing in any one of three substates; therefore, according to Table 8.3 both q and η vanish. The same argument applies to the 2-fold degenerate e orbitals. Thus any distribution of electrons among the t_2 and e orbitals gives $q = \eta = 0$ provided the t_2 and e orbitals retain their 3- and 2-fold degeneracies respectively; a nonvanishing contribution to q or η requires a further reduction in symmetry. Similar considerations apply to p electrons.

The case of an ion surrounded by ligands represents a much more complicated situation than that of a group of electrons occupying a set of specific orbitals.

In the first place we must take into account the effect of the closed shells. Although there are no direct contributions to the quadrupole splitting from closed shells, they are nevertheless sometimes polarized by valence electrons, and the ensuing distortion in the charge distribution alters the electric-field gradient at the nucleus. This effect is taken into account by the Sternheimer factor $(1-R)$ with $0<R<1$ (INGALLS, 1964). Another contribution to the quadrupole splitting comes from the charges on the ligands whose effect is also modified by a second Sternheimer factor $(1-\gamma_\infty)$ which may have values lying between 10 and 100. It is therefore customary to write

$$q = (1-R)q_v + (1-\gamma_\infty)q_l,$$
$$q\eta = (1-R)(q\eta)_v + (1-\gamma_\infty)(q\eta)_l$$

(8.1.21)

in which q_v and $(q\eta)_v$ are the contributions from valence electrons while q_l $(q\eta)_l$ are associated with the ligand charges.

· The special cases of interest in heme proteins are Fe^{2+} $(S=0,2)$ and Fe^{3+} $(S=\frac{1}{2},\frac{5}{2})$. If, at first, we adopt a strict crystal field approach, then, for $S=0$, each of the orbitals d_{xy}, d_{zx}, and d_{yz} is doubly occupied, and hence both q_v and $(q\eta)_v$ vanish. For $S=\frac{1}{2}$, d_{xy} and d_{zx} are doubly occupied while d_{yz} is singly occupied (Section 6.2). Hence

$$q_v = \tfrac{2}{7}\langle r^{-3}\rangle_{3d},$$

$(S=\frac{1}{2})$ $\qquad (q\eta)_v = \tfrac{6}{7}\langle r^{-3}\rangle_{3d},$ (8.1.22)

$$[q_v^2 + \tfrac{1}{3}(q\eta)_v^2]^{\frac{1}{2}} = \tfrac{4}{7}\langle r^{-3}\rangle_{3d}.$$

Finally, for $S=\frac{5}{2}$, each d orbital is singly occupied and again both q_v and $(q\eta)_v$ vanish. For $S=2$, the first five electrons occupy each of the d orbitals giving no net contribution to q_v or $(q\eta)_v$; the sixth electron is assumed to be in d_{xy}, which according to the interpretation of ESR experiments on ferrihemoglobin azide (Section 6.2), lies lowest. In that case

$$q_v = \tfrac{4}{7}\langle r^{-3}\rangle_{3d},$$

$(S=2)$ $\qquad (q\eta)_v = 0,$ (8.1.23)

$$[q_v^2 + \tfrac{1}{3}(q\eta)_v^2]^{\frac{1}{2}} = \tfrac{4}{7}\langle r^{-3}\rangle_{3d}.$$

From (8.1.22) and (8.1.23) it is seen that the valence part of the quadrupole splitting in low-spin ferric and high-spin ferrous hemoglobin should be the same.

For the ligand contribution—again on a purely crystal field basis—we note that the tetragonal and rhombic components of the crystal field can be written as in (5.3.1) and (5.3.2):

$$V_t + V_r = B_2^0(3z^2 - r^2) + B_2^2(x^2 - y^2),$$

in which higher-order terms have been neglected. Therefore

$$eq_l = V_{zz} = 4B_2^0,$$
$$e(q\eta)_l = V_{xx} - V_{yy} = 4B_2^2.$$

(8.1.24)

It is seen that the tetragonal field does not contribute to η, while the rhombic field does not contribute to q. From the matrix elements of V_t and V_r within the basis set of the $3d$ orbitals, we also find that

$$\delta = \tfrac{6}{7} e \langle r^2 \rangle_{3d} B_2^0 ,$$

$$\mu = \tfrac{4}{7} e \langle r^2 \rangle_{3d} B_2^2 \tag{8.1.25}$$

where δ and μ are the tetragonal and rhombic splittings respectively. Combining (8.1.24) with (8.1.25)

$$q_l = \frac{14\,\delta}{3\,e^2 \langle r^2 \rangle_{3d}} ,$$

$$(q\eta)_l = \frac{7\,\mu}{e^2 \langle r^2 \rangle_{3d}} . \tag{8.1.26}$$

The valence and ligand contributions to the quadrupole splitting can also be examined from the viewpoint of molecular orbital theory. For the valence part we sum the contributions from each valence orbital—$3d$ and $4p$ in Fe—weighted according to the calculated occupation numbers. The ligand contribution is given by

$$q_l = \sum_{i=1}^{N} Z_i \frac{3\cos^2 \theta_i - 1}{r_i^3}$$

$$(q\eta)_l = \sum_{i=1}^{N} Z_i \frac{3\sin^2 \theta_i \cos 2\phi_i}{r_i^3} \tag{8.1.27}$$

where Z_i is the charge on the i-th ligand and $(r_i, \theta_i, \varphi_i)$ its coordinates.

8.1.3 Magnetic Hyperfine Interactions

The third important type of interaction which enters into the interpretation of Mossbauer spectra is the interaction of the nucleus with a magnetic field. The field may be due to external sources or it may be produced internally as a result of various electronic configurations. In either case, the Hamiltonian for the magnetic interaction has the form

$$\mathcal{H}_m = -\boldsymbol{\mu} \cdot \boldsymbol{H} = -g_n \beta_n \boldsymbol{I} \cdot \boldsymbol{H} = -\gamma \hbar \boldsymbol{I} \cdot \boldsymbol{H}, \tag{8.1.28}$$

in which $\boldsymbol{\mu}$ and $\boldsymbol{I}$ are the nuclear magnetic moment and spin operators respectively; β_n is the nuclear Bohr magneton (5.05×10^{-24} ergs/G), γ is the gyromagnetic ratio and g_n is the nuclear g factor. If the z axis is taken along the direction of the magnetic field, the eigenvalues of $\mathcal{H}_m$ are

$$E_m = -g_n \beta_n m_I H. \tag{8.1.29}$$

Each nuclear level is therefore split into $(2I+1)$ substates so that for ^{57}Fe, the ground state $(I=\tfrac{1}{2})$ and the excited state are each split into 2 and 4 substates, respectively. These are the nuclear Zeeman levels. The most prominent transitions between $I=\tfrac{1}{2}$ and $I=\tfrac{3}{2}$ are those for which $\Delta m_I = 0$ or ± 1; a 6-line spectrum results. When the magnetic field has an arbitrary orientation relative to some chosen coordinate system which might be, for example, the principal axes of the EFG tensor, the Hamiltonian (8.1.28) becomes

$$\mathcal{H}_m = -\gamma \hbar H [I_x \sin\theta\cos\varphi + I_y \sin\theta\sin\varphi + I_z \cos\theta], \qquad (8.1.30)$$

where θ and φ are the polar and azimuth angles respectively. The matrix elements are readily calculated by converting the cartesian components of I to a spherical basis; the results are given in Table 8.4.

Table 8.4. *Matrix elements of the magnetic interaction Hamiltonian* (8.1.30)

$$I_g = \frac{1}{2}, \qquad -\gamma_g \hbar H = a$$

$\mathcal{H}_m$	$\frac{1}{2}$	$-\frac{1}{2}$
$\frac{1}{2}$	$\frac{a}{2}\cos\theta$	$\frac{a}{2}\sin\theta e^{-i\varphi}$
$-\frac{1}{2}$	$\frac{a}{2}\sin\theta e^{i\varphi}$	$-\frac{a}{2}\cos\theta$

$$I_e = \frac{3}{2} \qquad -\gamma_e \hbar H = b$$

$\mathcal{H}_m$	$\frac{3}{2}$	$-\frac{1}{2}$	$-\frac{3}{2}$	$\frac{1}{2}$
$\frac{3}{2}$	$\frac{3b}{2}\cos\theta$			$\frac{\sqrt{3}b}{2}\sin\theta e^{-i\varphi}$
$-\frac{1}{2}$		$-\frac{b}{2}\cos\theta$	$\frac{\sqrt{3}b}{2}\sin\theta e^{-i\varphi}$	$b\sin\theta e^{i\varphi}$
$-\frac{3}{2}$		$\frac{\sqrt{3}b}{2}\sin\theta e^{i\varphi}$	$-\frac{3b}{2}\cos\theta$	
$\frac{1}{2}$	$\frac{\sqrt{3}b}{2}\sin\theta e^{i\varphi}$	$b\sin\theta e^{-i\varphi}$		$\frac{b}{2}\cos\theta$

The magnetic hyperfine interaction may be described in terms of an effective magnetic field which has its origin in electronic motions. Such a field is defined as the expectation value of an operator, H_e, given by

$$H_e = -2\beta \sum_i \left[\left(\frac{l_i}{r_i^3} - \frac{s_i}{r_i^3} + 3\frac{r_i(s_i \cdot r_i)}{r_i^5} \right) + \frac{8\pi}{3} s_i \delta(r_i) \right], \qquad (8.1.31)$$

where s_i and l_i are the one-electron spin and orbital-angular momentum operators respectively. The first term in (8.1.31) is due to orbital currents; the next two, taken together, constitute the dipolar contribution and the last term, containing the δ function, is the Fermi contact interaction. The first three terms give nonvanishing contributions only for electrons with $l \neq 0$, in which case the contact term is zero. On the other hand, the field produced by s electrons is due entirely to the contact term. The summation is taken over all unpaired electrons; β is the (electronic) Bohr magneton.

Despite the fact that d orbitals vanish at the nucleus, there is an important indirect effect which gives rise to a large contribution from the Fermi contact term. This comes about as a result of exchange interactions between the d electron system and s electrons. The interaction depends on whether the spin of an s electron is parallel or antiparallel to the spin of the electronic state associated with the d^n configuration. In consequence, the radial charge distribution of s electrons with α spin $(m_s = \frac{1}{2})$ differs somewhat from that of s electrons with β spin $(m_s = -\frac{1}{2})$. The contact term in (8.1.31) can then be written (after integration of the δ function)

$$H_c = \frac{16\pi}{3} \beta s \left[\sum |\psi_\alpha(0)|^2 - \sum |\psi_\beta(0)|^2 \right], \tag{8.1.32}$$

where $\psi_\alpha(0)$ and $\psi_\beta(0)$ are the wave functions at the nucleus of s electrons with α and β spin respectively. Such an imbalance in s electron density (polarization effect), though seemingly quite small, may nevertheless produce magnetic fields at the nucleus of $300 - 500 \, \mathrm{kG}$. A formally equivalent approach is to regard the high magnetic field at the nucleus in d electron systems as arising from a mixing of the d^n configuration with excited configurations which contain unpaired s electrons.

These effects are difficult to express quantitatively; it is therefore customary to incorporate a semi-empirical parameter, κ, into the Fermi contact term so that the magnetic hyperfine interaction is written

$$\mathcal{H}_m = 2\beta\gamma\hbar I \cdot \sum \left[\frac{(l_i - s_i)}{r_i^3} + 3 \frac{r_i(s_i \cdot r_i)}{r_i^5} - \frac{\kappa s_i}{r_i^3} \right]$$

with κ, for d^n configurations, approximately equal to 0.35. In the spin Hamiltonian formalism, $\mathcal{H}_m$ may be recast into

$$\mathcal{H}_m = A_x I_x S_x + A_y I_y S_y + A_z I_z S_z \tag{8.1.33}$$

in which A_x, A_y and A_z are known as the principal components of the magnetic hyperfine coupling tensor; they may or may not all be alike, depending on the crystal symmetry. If it is sufficient to regard the hyperfine interaction as due almost entirely to core polarization, the contact term will dominate and (8.1.33) can be approximated by an isotropic spin Hamiltonian

$$\mathcal{H}_m = A I \cdot S,$$
$$A = -2\beta\gamma\hbar\kappa \langle r^{-3} \rangle. \tag{8.1.34}$$

In Mossbauer spectroscopy both the ground and the excited states of $^{57}\mathrm{Fe}$ interact with the internal field. The expressions given above apply to either state though the coupling constants in the two states differ both in magnitude and sign (Table 8.1).

The isomer shift and the quadrupole splitting are not well defined for time intervals less than the lifetime of the excited state, τ, which is 1.41×10^{-7} sec. The latter can therefore be regarded as the characteristic time for these two parameters. In the case of the magnetic hyperfine interaction there are two additional characteristic times. One is the period of the Lamor precession, τ_L, of the nuclear magnetic moment in the effective internal magnetic field generated by the surrounding electrons. The precession time is inversely proportional to the magnetic field

$$\tau_L = \frac{2\pi}{\gamma H} \approx \frac{h}{E} \tag{8.1.35}$$

where E is the magnetic hyperfine splitting. The second characteristic time is associated with the random fluctuations suffered by the electronic spins. The mean time between successive changes in spin orientation (space quantization) of the magnetic electrons defines a relaxation time, τ_R. The two most important contributions to τ_R are spin-lattice (T_1) and spin-spin (T_2) relaxations. In substances containing a low concentration of paramagnetic species separated by large distances (as in hemoglobin), T_2 becomes long compared with T_1; τ_R is therefore determined almost entirely by the spin-lattice relaxation. The latter requires a spin-orbit interaction in order to couple electronic spins with phonon modes of the lattice. Therefore, in the absence of orbital angular momentum, relaxation times are relatively long ($\sim 10^{-8}$ sec); a reduction in temperature also increases T_1 and hence τ_R.

We must now consider the relative magnitudes of τ, τ_L and τ_R; the discussion is confined to paramagnetic materials. In the first place, if $\tau \ll \tau_L$, i. e. the nuclear excited state decays before completion of a Larmor precession period, it will not be possible to establish a well-defined magnetic hyperfine structure. This sets a lower limit for the effective internal magnetic field which, according to (8.1.35), is about 10 kG for ^{57}Fe. Since internal fields are usually far in excess of this value, this condition is not restrictive.

The relative magnitude of τ_L and τ_R is a critical factor in determining whether magnetic hyperfine interactions can occur. If $\tau_L \ll \tau_R$, the nuclear magnetic moment is capable of following fluctuations in the electronic magnetic moment; one may then expect to observe line broadening and perhaps even a fully resolved hyperfine spectrum. In the opposite limit, $\tau_L \gg \tau_R$, the fluctuations in the spins are rapid enough to average out the effective magnetic field at the nucleus and there is therefore no hyperfine structure. There is also the intermediate case when $\tau_R \sim \tau_L$; this case usually results in a complicated spectrum in which the number of lines, their positions, intensities, and widths depend on specific details (BRADFORD and MARSHALL, 1966; WEISSBLUTH, 1971).

When both quadrupole and magnetic interactions are present, the spectra become quite complex. In a few special cases, such as when the direction of the magnetic field (z axis) coincides with one of the principal axes of the EFG tensor, it is possible to give closed expressions for the combined interaction. Then

$$\left(I_g = \frac{1}{2}\right) \qquad E = \pm \frac{\gamma_g h H}{2}, \tag{8.1.36}$$

$$\left(I_e = \frac{3}{2}\right) \qquad E = \begin{cases} \dfrac{\gamma_e \hbar H}{2} \pm \dfrac{e^2 q Q}{4}\left[\left(1 + \dfrac{4\gamma_e \hbar H}{e^2 q Q}\right)^2 + \dfrac{\eta^2}{3}\right]^{\frac{1}{2}}, \\[3mm] -\dfrac{\gamma_e \hbar H}{2} \pm \dfrac{e^2 q Q}{4}\left[\left(1 - \dfrac{4\gamma_e \hbar H}{e^2 q Q}\right)^2 + \dfrac{\eta^2}{3}\right]^{\frac{1}{2}}. \end{cases} \qquad (8.1.37)$$

The spectrum may contain as many as 8 lines with various intensities, so that only under very favorable conditions will such a spectrum be resolved.

In paramagnetic substances, relatively weak magnetic fields may have a profound effect on the hyperfine spectrum. This may be seen in the following manner: with no external magnetic field present, the electronic and nuclear angular momenta are coupled by the magnetic hyperfine interaction. Because electronic magnetic moments are of the order of a thousand times greater than nuclear moments, the effective magnetic field at the position of an electron is smaller—in inverse ratio to the magnetic moments— than the field at the nucleus. Typically, effective fields seen by $3d$ electrons are less than 100 G. It is therefore possible to decouple the electronic and nuclear angular momenta by the application of an external magnetic field of several hundred gauss. S and I then precess independently about the external field. Under these circumstances the electronic spins are kept in alignment and, through the polarization effect, induce a contact interaction which, as we have seen, can result in effective magnetic fields at the nucleus of several hundred thousand gauss. The hyperfine structure in the Mossbauer spectrum is then readily resolved. We see, then, that a small external field may overcome the effects of fast relaxations which would otherwise wipe out the magnetic hyperfine structure. In an electronic state in which the spins are all paired ($S=0$), the field can interact only with the nuclear magnetic moment to produce Zeeman splitting of the nuclear levels. To resolve such splittings high fields ($>50\,\mathrm{kG}$) are required.

The transition between the excited state $I_e = \frac{3}{2}$ and the ground state $I_g = \frac{1}{2}$ is of the magnetic dipole type (M 1), and is therefore governed by the selection rule

$$\Delta m = 0, +1.$$

The intensities of the six allowed transitions are proportional to

$$\begin{pmatrix} \frac{3}{2} & 1 & \frac{1}{2} \\ -m_e & M & m_g \end{pmatrix}^2 F_L^M(\theta)$$

with

$$-m_e + M + m_g = 0.$$

The 3-j symbol represents the coupling of the angular momenta $I_e = \frac{3}{2}$ and $I_g = \frac{1}{2}$ through the magnetic dipole radiation field for which $L=1$. m_e, M, and m_g are projection quantum numbers for I_e, L, and I_g respectively. $F_L^M(\theta)$ is an angular factor:

$$F_1^0(\theta) = \tfrac{3}{2}\sin^2\theta,$$
$$F_1^{\pm 1}(\theta) = \tfrac{3}{4}(1+\cos^2\theta)$$

in which θ is the angle between the axis of quantization and the direction of observation. The relative intensities are shown in Table 8.5.

Table 8.5. *Relative intensities of Mossbauer transitions in* ^{57}Fe

m_e ($I_e = \frac{3}{2}$)	m_g ($I_g = \frac{1}{2}$)	Relative Intensity	Average Relative Intensity
$\frac{3}{2}$	$\frac{1}{2}$	$\frac{3}{4}(1+\cos^2\theta)$	1
$\frac{1}{2}$	$\frac{1}{2}$	$\sin^2\theta$	$\frac{2}{3}$
$-\frac{1}{2}$	$\frac{1}{2}$	$\frac{1}{4}(1+\cos^2\theta)$	$\frac{1}{3}$
$\frac{1}{2}$	$-\frac{1}{2}$	$\frac{1}{4}(1+\cos^2\theta)$	$\frac{1}{3}$
$-\frac{1}{2}$	$-\frac{1}{2}$	$\sin^2\theta$	$\frac{2}{3}$
$-\frac{3}{2}$	$-\frac{1}{2}$	$\frac{3}{4}(1+\cos^2\theta)$	1

In the absence of any perturbations the single transition between $I_e = \frac{3}{2}$ and $I_g = \frac{1}{2}$ has a relative intensity given by the sum of the intensities for the six allowed transitions. This sum is seen to be independent of θ. When a quadrupole interaction is present, the excited state with $I_e = \frac{3}{2}$ becomes a doublet while the ground state with $I_g = \frac{1}{2}$ remains unaffected. The relative intensities of the two possible transitions, $\pm\frac{3}{2}(I_e = \frac{3}{2}) \rightarrow \pm\frac{1}{2}(I_g = \frac{1}{2})$ and $\pm\frac{1}{2}(I_e = \frac{3}{2}) \rightarrow \pm\frac{1}{2}(I_g = \frac{1}{2})$, become identical. Finally, when a magnetic field is applied the degeneracies are completely removed and the six transitions averaged over all directions have intensities in the ratio $3:2:1:1:2:3$.

8.2 Mossbauer Spectra of Hemoglobin

A considerably body of Mossbauer data now exists on heme proteins (LANG and MARSHALL, 1966; MALING and WEISSBLUTH, 1969; BEARDEN and DUNHAM, 1970; DEBRUNNER, 1970; LANG, 1970; WINTER *et al.*, 1972). Since native hemoglobin contains only 0.0074% of ^{57}Fe, it is usually necessary to work with samples that have been isotopically enriched in ^{57}Fe. This is particularly important for studies of magnetic hyperfine structure which contain many lines of low signal amplitude. Nevertheless, it is often feasible to obtain satisfactory spectra with unenriched samples in the form of either lyophilized powder or concentrated (30%) frozen solutions. The conditions under which Mossbauer experiments are conducted, in common with other methods e.g. ESR, are therefore far from physiological, especially in anhydrous samples in which changes in conformation and spin are likely to occur.

Data on quadrupole splittings and isomer shifts are summarized in Table 8.6. The various compounds can also be classified according to their position on a plot of isomer shift (δ) vs. quadrupole splitting (ΔE) (MALING and WEISSBLUTH, 1969). Three main groups are found:

a) $\delta \approx 1.0$ mm/sec $- \Delta E \approx 2.0$ mm/sec: the only compound in this region is deoxyhemoglobin;

b) $\delta \approx 0.2$ mm/sec $- \Delta E \approx 2.0$ mm/sec: this is the largest group, containing oxyhemoglobin, methemoglobin, ferrihemoglobin hydroxide and azide. Ferrihemoglobin cyanide also lies close to this region, though it has a somewhat smaller quadrupole splitting;

c) $\delta \approx 0.2$ mm/sec $- \Delta E \approx 0.3$ mm/sec: carboxyhemoglobin is the only compound in this region.

We shall now give a brief description of the Mossbauer spectra of several
hemoglobin derivatives. Considering first the ferrous derivatives (Fig. 8.1), the
spectrum of oxyhemoglobin $(S=0)$ consists of a symmetric doublet whose
quadrupole coupling constant has been found to be negative (LANG and
MARSHALL, 1966). Carboxyhemoglobin might be expected to exhibit a spectrum
similar to that of oxyhemoglobin since it, too, is ferrous and low-spin. This is
so for the isomer shift but the quadrupole splitting is far smaller—by a factor
of about 5. In deoxyhemoglobin $(S=2)$, the quadrupole splitting is comparable,
though slightly larger than that of oxyhemoglobin; however, the isomer shift is
larger by a factor of $3-4$. The latter appears to be a distinctive feature of high-
spin ferrous compounds and is often used as a means of identification. In all
three ferrous compounds a reduction in temperature produces a more intense
absorption and an increase in the quadrupole splitting by about $10-15\%$ as
the temperature is lowered from $200 °K$ to about $4 °K$. However, there is no
evidence of any magnetic hyperfine structure even at the lowest temperatures.

The isomer shifts and quadrupole splittings of ferric proteins lie in the same
range as oxyhemoglobin. An exception occurs in ferrihemoglobin fluoride which
has an unusually small splitting of about 0.6 mm/sec in frozen solution, though
in powder form $\Delta E = 2.0$ mm/sec as in other ferric proteins. At sufficiently low
temperatures, the spectra of ferric hemoglobins become broad and quite com-

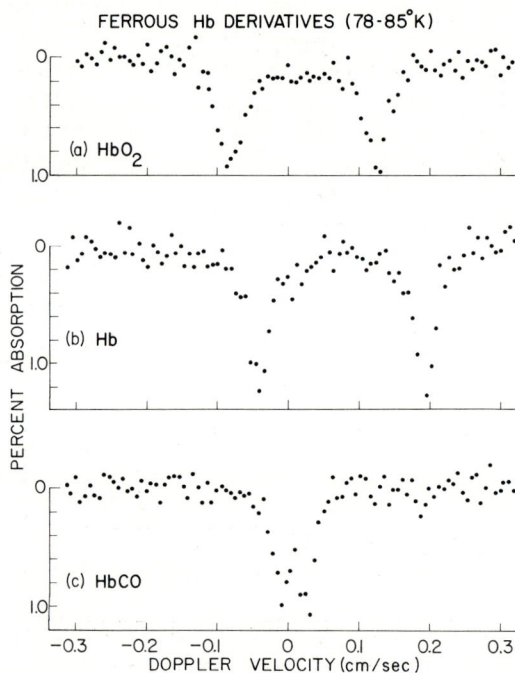

Fig. 8.1 a—c. Mossbauer spectra in a) oxyhemoglobin, b) deoxyhemoglobin and c) carboxyhemoglobin at 78—85 °K (MALING and WEISSBLUTH, 1969)

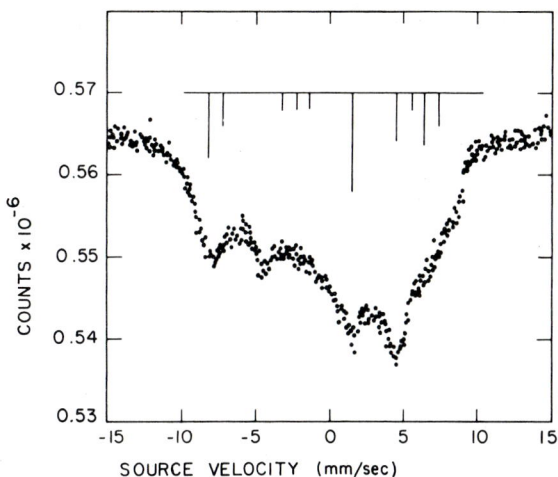

Fig. 8.2. Mossbauer spectrum and predicted line pattern in methemoglobin, pH 6.0, at 1.2 °K (LANG and MARSHALL, 1966)

plicated (Figs. 8.2 and 8.3) as a result of magnetic hyperfine interactions. In some cases, as in ferrihemoglobin fluoride, the effects are observable even at moderate temperature (~ 200 °K). Such behavior might be expected in a high-spin ferric system in which the ground state is an orbital singlet ($L = 0$). Spin-orbit coupling

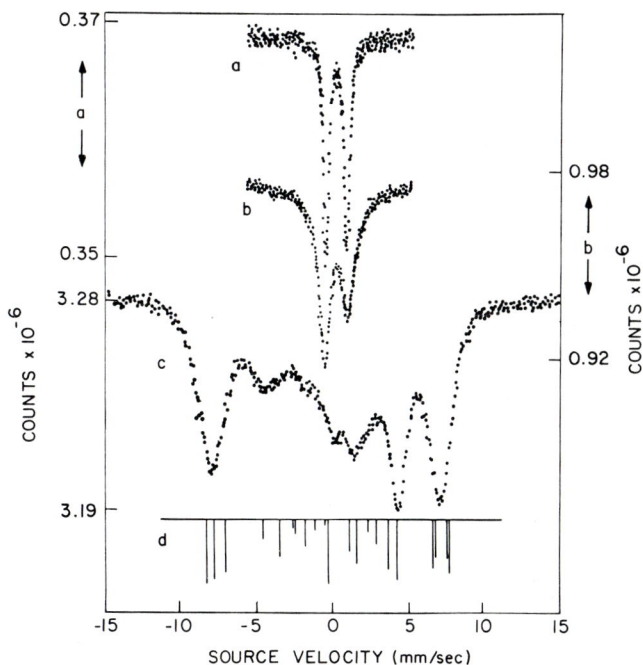

Fig. 8.3 a—d. Mossbauer spectra in ferrihemoglobin cyanide at a) 195 °K, b) 77 °K and c) 4 °K. The predicted line pattern is shown in d) (LANG, 1967)

can then occur only in higher orders. The electronic system is therefore well-insulated from the lattice and we would anticipate low rates of spin-lattice relaxation. Yet in methemoglobin, another high-spin ferric compound, the magnetic hyperfine interaction has a different temperature dependence, and it appears that the spin-lattice relaxation rate is far greater than in the fluoride. In the low-spin ferric derivatives it is necessary to reduce the temperature to about 4°K before any evidence of magnetic hyperfine interaction can be observed. The application of an external magnetic field has been found to be a useful expedient in analysis of the magnetic hyperfine interaction; this will be discussed in the next section.

Some additional features of Mossbauer spectra are the following: the spectra are insensitive to the species from which the hemoglobin has been derived, despite differences in amino-acid composition. Mutant varieties of human hemoglobin which differ drastically in their physiological behavior nevertheless produce almost the same Mossbauer spectra. These results, and others, suggest what is expected on general grounds, that the Mossbauer spectra are primarily influenced by the local environment in the vicinity of the iron atom. It should further be kept in mind that hemoglobins tend to exist as mixtures of high- and low-spin states so that characterization by means of a spin state is, at best, only an approximation.

8.3 Theoretical Interpretation and Discussion

The quantitative interpretation of isomer shifts in heme proteins appears to be difficult (WEISSBLUTH and MALING, 1967), and it has not progressed significantly beyond the ideas outlined in Section 8.1.1. The discussion below is therefore confined to the quadrupole splitting and the magnetic hyperfine interaction.

8.3.1 Quadrupole Splitting

We first consider the predictions based entirely on crystal field theory. It has already been shown (Section 8.1.12) that there can be no contributions to the quadrupole splitting (ΔE) from electrons residing in the 5-fold degenerate $3d$ shell, nor is there any splitting in cubic symmetry. Only when the symmetry is reduced still further do we get non-vanishing contributions. In a few cases it is possible to compare the crystal field predictions (Section 8.1.2) with experimental values of ΔE (Table 8.6). It is seen, for example, that oxy- and carboxyhemoglobin, both with an electronic configuration t_2^6 and $S=0$, should have no splitting; experimentally, both derivatives are observed to have completely different, non-vanishing values of ΔE. Methemoglobin ($t_2^3 e^2, S=\frac{5}{2}$) should also have no splitting theoretically, yet the experimental value is quite large. Oxy- and deoxyhemoglobin have almost the same value of ΔE, whereas the predicted values are quite different. Clearly, crystal field theory in its simplest form is quite inadequate for the interpretation of quadrupole splittings. It is therefore of interest to inquire whether any improvement in interpretation may be achieved through the use of molecular orbital theory in which covalency

Table 8.6. *Quadrupole splittings (ΔE) and isomer shifts (δ) for hemoglobin derivatives; S = frozen solution, P = lyophilized powder (*LANG *and* MARSHALL, *1966;* MALING *and* WEISSBLUTH, *1969)*

Derivative		Spin	ΔE mm/sec	δ mm/sec
Oxyhemoglobin	(HbO$_2$)	0	1.9 − 2.3	0.20 − 0.31
Carboxyhemoglobin	(HbCO)	0	0.3 − 0.4	0.18 − 0.27
Deoxyhemoglobin	(Hb)	2	2.1 − 2.5	0.90 − 1.1
Ferrihemoglobin				
cyanide	(HbCN)	$\frac{1}{2}$	1.2 − 1.4	0.16 − 0.22
azide	(HbN$_3$)	$\frac{1}{2}$	2.0 − 2.3	0.15 − 0.25
hydroxide	(HbOH)	$\frac{1}{2} - \frac{5}{2}$	1.6 − 1.9	0.18 − 0.2
fluoride	(HbF)	$\frac{5}{2}$	0.6 (S) 2.0 (P)	0.9
Methemoglobin	(HbH$_2$O)	$\frac{5}{2}$	1.9 − 2.1	0.14 − 0.26

effects are included as an intrinsic feature of the calculation, in contrast to crystal field theory, which completely neglects covalency.

The computation of quadrupole splittings on the basis of molecular orbital theory has been outlined in Section 8.1. If we call f_d and f_p the electronic populations in $3d$ and $4p$ orbitals respectively, then

$$q_v = \sum_d f_d q_d + \sum_p f_p q_p,$$

$$(q\eta)_v = \sum_d f_d (q\eta)_d + \sum_p f_p (q\eta)_p. \tag{8.3.1}$$

The quantities q_d, q_p, η_d and η_p are given in Table 8.3; f_d and f_p are taken from the calculations of ZERNER et al. (1966) (ZGK) on iron porphins. Table 7.5 lists the values for selected prophins. Similarly, q_l and $(q\eta)_l$ are given by (8.1.27), in which the coordinates and charges are those of the ZGK calculation (Tables 7.3 and 7.6). It is then possible to compute ΔE by means of (8.1.21) and (8.1.15). Such a computation was carried out by WEISSBLUTH and MALING (1967) with the following conclusions: The molecular orbital approach appears to be capable of distinguishing between oxy- and carboxyhemoglobin, though both are ferrous low-spin compounds, and satisfactorily predicts that oxyhemoglobin will have a large quadrupole splitting relative to carboxyhemoglobin. The computation also shows that the quadrupole coupling constant in oxyhemoglobin is positive; this is of opposite sign to the results of experiments in external magnetic fields (LANG and MARSHALL, 1966). The splittings in oxy- and deoxyhemoglobin are predicted to be nearly the same, in agreement with experiment. Ferric high-spin compounds are predicted to have a large quadrupole splitting but with a negative quadrupole coupling constant. The large splitting is verified experimentally in methemoglobin, for example, and the negative quadrupole coupling constant agrees with that obtained by LANG and MARSHALL (1966), who based their conclusion on a totally different calculation. However, there does not seem to be any experimental information with which to compare the sign of the calculated coupling constant. Finally, the predicted similarity of the splittings in ferric high- and low-spin compounds is also borne out by experiments. It appears, then, that the molecular orbital approach, when compared with that of crystal field theory, provides the more rational basis for the interpretation of quadrupole splittings, though, clearly, difficulties still remain. Nevertheless, it would be reasonable to conclude that the electric field gradient at the nucleus is highly sensitive to delocalization or covalency effects and it is only when such effects are taken into account in a detailed fashion that we can hope to construct a coherent theory.

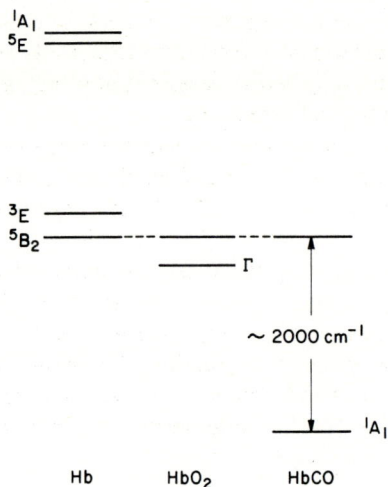

Fig. 8.4. Lowest energy states in deoxyhemoglobin (Hb), oxyhemoglobin (HbO$_2$) and carboxyhemoglobin (HbCO) (TRAUTWEIN et al., 1970)

Much of the information concerning the electronic states of ferric hemoglobins has been deduced from electron-spin resonance experiments. Such experiments cannot be performed with the ferrous derivatives and as a result our knowledge of their electronic states is far less detailed. An attempt to employ Mossbauer data for this purpose was made by EICHER and TRAUTWEIN (1970) and by TRAUTWEIN et al. (1970). In particular, they concentrated on the temperature dependence of the quadrupole splitting in ferrous hemoglobins—an approach which is analogous to that based on the temperature dependence of the magnetic susceptibility. In D_{4h} symmetry, with some rhombic distortion, they deduce an energy level structure which is shown in Fig. 8.4. In deoxyhemoglobin, $^5B_2$ is the ground state; in oxyhemoglobin, the ground state (Γ) is regarded as a linear combination of ^3E (in Fe) and a triplet state in oxygen so as to give a net spin $S=0$. The ground state of carboxyhemoglobin ($^1A_1$) lies approximately 2000 cm^{-1} below that of oxyhemoglobin and it is conjectured that it is this difference in energy which accounts for the much greater affinity of hemoglobin for CO than for O$_2$.

8.3.2 Magnetic Hyperfine Interaction

Ferrous compounds do not exhibit any magnetic hyperfine structure. This is an expected result for the low-spin compounds with $S=0$. However, in deoxy-hemoglobin, with $S=2$, magnetic hyperfine interactions might conceivably occur. That they do not, even at low temperatures, might be attributed to a high relaxation rate as a result of spin-orbit coupling in the ground state. Also, since the unfilled $3d$ shell in ferrous systems contains an even number of electrons, Kramers' theorem does not apply. It is then possible for a crystal field of low symmetry to remove all degeneracies. If, then, the ground state is a singlet which does not mix significantly with higher states, it will have no magnetic moment and will therefore be unable to engage in magnetic interactions with the nucleus. We note that the considerations concerning the lack of magnetic hyperfine inter-actions in high-spin ferrous systems are essentially the same as those associated with the lack of electron-spin resonance.

LANG and MARSHALL (1966) made effective use of external magnetic fields in the analysis of Mossbauer spectra. We shall describe their method in the form in which it was applied to high-spin $(S=\frac{5}{2})$ ferric systems.

We have seen that the magnetic field at the electronic positions, due to the magnetic moment of ^{57}Fe, is quite small—less than 100 gauss. Therefore, an external field of several hundred gauss is sufficient to decouple the electronic and nuclear spins. It is then justifiable to diagonalize the electronic Hamiltonian without reference to the nuclear interaction. The resulting eigenstates together with the nuclear eigenstates then constitute a zero-order basis set for the computation of the magnetic hyperfine interaction. The electronic-spin Hamiltonian (Section 6.3) is given by

$$\mathscr{H}(S) = D\left[S_z^2 - \tfrac{1}{3}S(S+1)\right] + 2\beta\, \boldsymbol{H} \cdot \boldsymbol{S} \qquad (8.3.2)$$

and the solutions are shown in Fig. 6.5. Since the value of D in hemoglobin is $6-10\ \mathrm{cm}^{-1}$ (Table 6.2), it is only the lowest doublet, effectively, which is occupied at $4\,°K$. An important consequence of such an uneven occupation is that the effective spin of the system is no longer $\frac{5}{2}$. A calculation of the expectation value of $\boldsymbol{S}$ reveals this feature.

If, at first, a very small magnetic field is applied along the symmetry axis $(H_z = H_{\parallel})$, the eigenfunctions of the Hamiltonian (6.3.25) are simply $|\pm\tfrac{1}{2}\rangle$. Then

$$\begin{aligned}
\langle S_z\rangle_+ &= \langle\tfrac{1}{2}|S_z|\tfrac{1}{2}\rangle = \tfrac{1}{2},\\
\langle S_z\rangle_- &= \langle-\tfrac{1}{2}|S_z|-\tfrac{1}{2}\rangle = -\tfrac{1}{2}.
\end{aligned} \qquad (8.3.3)$$

When the magnetic field is applied in the transverse direction $(H_\perp)$, the Hamiltonian assumes the form shown in (6.3.31). Thus, for $H_\perp = H_x$

$$\psi_\pm = \frac{1}{\sqrt{2}}\left[|\tfrac{1}{2}\rangle \pm |-\tfrac{1}{2}\rangle\right] \qquad (8.3.4)$$

and

$$\begin{aligned}
\langle S_x\rangle_+ &= \langle\psi_+|S_x|\psi_+\rangle = \tfrac{3}{2},\\
\langle S_x\rangle_- &= \langle\psi_-|S_x|\psi_-\rangle = -\tfrac{3}{2}
\end{aligned} \qquad (8.3.5)$$

where it must be remembered in the evaluation of (8.3.5) that $S=\frac{5}{2}$. The results for $\langle S_y \rangle$ are the same; for the expectation values of the spin we therefore have

$$|\langle S_\| \rangle| = \tfrac{1}{2}; \quad |\langle S_\perp \rangle| = \tfrac{3}{2}. \tag{8.3.6}$$

These results are also closely related to the fact that in the lowest doublet $g_\|=2$ and $g_\perp=6$. It is seen, then, that the spin properties of the electronic system depend very markedly on the direction of the applied field and that this feature is a direct consequence of the crystal field symmetry.

In polycrystalline materials, the heme planes of the various molecules are randomly oriented relative to an externally applied magnetic field. Nevertheless, as discussed in Section 6.5, the probability of the magnetic field lying in or near the heme plane (transverse direction) is very high. Quantitatively, the probability that the field makes an angle θ with the symmetry axis is proportional to $\sin\theta$. Therefore in a polycrystalline sample—the form in which most experiments are conducted—it is a good approximation to treat magnetic effects solely on the basis of $\langle S_\perp \rangle$.

When the magnetic field is increased, the values of $\langle S_\perp \rangle$ begin to deviate from $\pm\frac{3}{2}$. The reason for this (Section 6.5 and Fig. 6.6) is that the magnetic substates of the lowest Kramers doublet approach the magnetic substates of the next higher doublet. The magnetic field $(H_\perp)$ then mixes the wave functions so that the eigenstates are no longer given by (8.3.4). The detailed behavior may be deduced from the matrix elements listed in Table 6.7 or it may be seen qualitatively from Fig. 6.6. The net effect is summarized below:

	low H	high H
$\langle S_\perp \rangle_-$	$-\frac{3}{2}$	$-\frac{5}{2}$
$\langle S_\perp \rangle_+$	$+\frac{3}{2}$	$-\frac{3}{2}$

In terms of absolute values, $|\langle S_\perp \rangle_-|$ increases from $\frac{3}{2}$ to an asymptotic value of $\frac{5}{2}$ while $|\langle S_\perp \rangle_+|$ at first decreases from $\frac{3}{2}$ to zero and then increases to an asymptotic value of $\frac{3}{2}$.

With these considerations in mind, the Hamiltonian for the magnetic hyperfine interaction, in the presence of an external magnetic field, H, can be written

$$\mathcal{H}_g = A_g I \cdot \langle S \rangle - \gamma_g \hbar I \cdot H \tag{8.3.7}$$

for the nuclear ground state, and

$$\mathcal{H}_e = A_e I \cdot \langle S \rangle - \gamma_e \hbar I \cdot H + \frac{e^2 q Q}{4}\left[I_z^2 - \frac{5}{4} + \frac{\eta}{3}(I_x^2 - I_y^2) \right] \tag{8.3.8}$$

for the nuclear excited state. In (8.3.8), the quadrupole interaction with $I=\frac{3}{2}$ has been included. The second term in each Hamiltonian describes the direct interaction of the external magnetic field, H, with the nucleus. This is but a small contribution compared with the first term in which the magnetic field does not appear explicitly. Yet the field must be present in order to decouple the electronic and spin angular momenta. This leads to the replacement of the spin operator S by its expectation value $\langle S \rangle$ which, through the mechanism of core polarization, produces a magnetic field at the nucleus many times greater than the external field. We see, then, that the most important feature of (8.3.7) and (8.3.8) is the presence of $\langle S \rangle$, which is put equal to $\langle S_\perp \rangle$ for polycrystalline samples. Also, since the overall interaction is dominated by the contact term resulting from core polarization,

$$A_g = -2\beta\gamma_g\hbar\kappa\langle r^{-3}\rangle_{3d} \tag{8.3.9}$$

with a corresponding expression for A_e.

LANG and MARSHALL (1966) carried through this calculation on ferrihemo-globin fluoride with the assumption that the electronic relaxation time was slow according to the criteria of Section 8.1.3. Their findings can be summarized as follows. At low temperature and in a small magnetic field, which is effectively transverse, $\langle S_\perp \rangle_+$ and $\langle S_\perp \rangle_-$ each produce a six-line hyperfine spectrum. Since $|\langle S_\perp \rangle_+| = |\langle S_\perp \rangle_-|$, the two spectra superimpose. At higher fields, the above equality is no longer valid, and two separate six-line spectra are observed. The quantitative analysis of these spectra established the spin Hamiltonian parameters which were then used to predict the zero field spectrum. When compared with the experimental one, the fit was not good. Subsequently, an improved fit was obtained by taking into account the transferred hyperfine interaction with the fluorine and nitrogen nuclei.

In its basic features the analysis of the magnetic hyperfine structure of low-spin ferric hemoglobin proceeds along similar lines. The electronic structure is shown in Fig. 6.3. In this case, too, it is sufficient to consider only the lowest Kramers doublet since the next higher doublet is approximately $1000\,\mathrm{cm}^{-1}$ away. The constants A_1, B_1, and C_1 of the lowest doublet (6.2.1) are related to the g values of electron-spin resonance experiments by (6.2.7). It is therefore possible to apply external magnetic fields and to proceed as in the high-spin ferric case, though the details of the calculation will be entirely different. LANG and MARSHALL (1966) established relationship connecting the hyperfine param-eters to A_1, B_1, and C_1, and in this way obtained a fit to the Mossbauer spectrum of ferrihemoglobin azide at $4\,^\circ$K and $1.2\,^\circ$K without any adjustable parameters.

It is clear that a great deal of information is contained in the Mossbauer spectra of hemoglobin and its various derivatives, though extracting such infor-mation with confidence is quite another matter. This situation is not significantly different from other types of spectroscopy which are used more often in a semi-empirical fashion, in conjunction with other physical and chemical methods, for diagnostic purposes.

Chapter IX

Further Aspects

9.1 Diamagnetism of Oxyhemoglobin

Oxyhemoglobin is diamagnetic $(S=0)$. Assuming that the oxidation state is Fe^{2+} and the electronic configuration is t_2^6, the spin of the six $3d$ electrons will be paired and we should not expect any paramagnetism from this source. But the ground state of molecular oxygen is known to be a triplet $(S=1)$. Why, then, does oxyhemoglobin not exhibit paramagnetism attributable to the presence of O_2?

Various answers have been given to this question. GRIFFITH (1956) assumed that the axis of the oxygen molecule lies parallel to the heme plane:

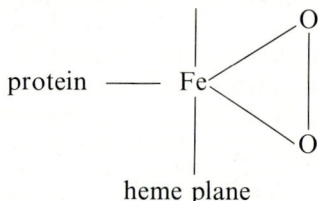

In such an orientation, covalent bonding between O_2 and the iron-porphyrin system has the effect of reducing the symmetry about the O—O axis. For the implication of the reduction in symmetry to be seen it must be recalled that the two (antibonding) molecular orbitals π_x^* and π_y^* of O_2 are normally degenerate. Each orbital contains a single electron, and the exchange energy favors a parallel alignment of the spins leading to $S=1$. Upon reduction of the symmetry about the O—O axis, π_x^* and π_y^* are no longer degenerate and the state with $S=1$ is not necessarily the one of lowest energy. GRIFFITH therefore assumed that in oxyhemoglobin, the valence state of O_2 is in a diamagnetic excited configuration. On this basis, a perpendicular orientation of the O—O axis relative to the heme plane would imply that the complex would tend to be paramagnetic.

The diamagnetism of oxyhemoglobin has also been regarded as arising from the configuration $Fe^{3+}O_2^-$. According to this view there is a net transfer of electronic charge from Fe to O_2. If it is assumed that the transfer takes place from a filled t_2 shell without any further electronic rearrangements, an appropriate description of the electronic state of iron would be Fe^{3+} (t_2^5) with $S=\frac{1}{2}$; at the same time the oxygen molecule would become O_2^-, also with $S=\frac{1}{2}$. The two unpaired spins can then couple to produce a diamagnetic state $(S=0)$. The fact that oxyhemoglobin has an isomer shift and quadrupole splitting very similar to that of the ferric compounds (MALING and WEISSBLUTH, 1969) is consistent with this hypothesis. Further support is derived from absorption spectra and the acid dissociation constant (WEISS, 1964), optical spectra (WITTENBERG *et al.*, 1970), and X-ray fluorescence spectra (KOSTER, 1972). A rather different approach was developed by TRAUTWEIN *et al.* (1970), who concluded that the diamagnetism of oxyhemoglobin arises from the coupling of two triplet states ($S = 1$), one being an intermediate state in Fe^{2+} and the other the normal ground state of O_2.

It is of interest in this connection to note that the calculations of ZERNER *et al.* (1966) show that there is no clear distinction, on the basis of net charge on Fe, between ferric and ferrous compounds, although among the iron porphins that were calculated, the one having O_2 as an axial ligand (with the O—O axis parallel to the porphin plane) shows the largest transfer of charge from Fe to O_2. It might therefore be said that in a system in which there is extensive delocalization of charge, the classification into ferrous and ferric is probably too simplistic and that the real situation is considerably more subtle.

The calculations of GRIFFITH (1956) and those of ZERNER *et al.* (1966) favor an orientation of the oxygen molecule with the O—O axis parallel to the heme plane as opposed to a perpendicular attachment. However, intermediate orientations are not ruled out, and indeed it was PAULING (1949, 1964) who first proposed an arrangement with the O—O axis inclined at 60° to the heme plane:

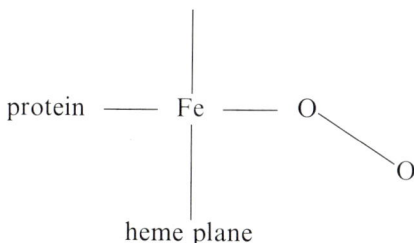

9.2 The Jahn-Teller Effect and Cooperativity in Hemoglobin

Some aspects of the Jahn-Teller effect have been described in Section 5.7. We now wish to extend that discussion with the aim of examining the possibility that the Jahn-Teller effect may have a bearing on the cooperativity of hemoglobin.

For a system of electrons and nuclei

$$\mathscr{H} = \mathscr{H}_n(Q_k, P_k) + \mathscr{H}_o(q, p) + V(q, Q_k). \tag{9.1}$$

$\mathscr{H}_n$ is the nuclear Hamiltonian for which it is sufficient to adopt a harmonic approximation

$$\mathscr{H}_n = \sum_k \left(\frac{P_k^2}{2m} + \frac{1}{2} m \omega_k^2 Q_k^2 \right). \tag{9.2}$$

The quantities Q_k are the coordinates of the normal modes whose frequencies are ω_k and whose conjugate momenta are P_k; m is the nuclear mass (for simplicity we assume all nuclei to be of the same kind). $\mathcal{H}_0(q,p)$, in which q and p are electronic coordinates and momenta, is the Hamiltonian for the electronic motion when the nuclei are clamped in their equilibrium positions, i. e. when all $Q_k=0$. The last term, $V(q,Q_k)$, represents a coupling between the electronic and nuclear motions; it arises as a consequence of the fact that the electronic eigenvalues and eigenfunctions depend on the positions of the nuclei. To first order in Q_k

$$\mathcal{H} = \mathcal{H}_0(q,p) + \sum_k \left[\left(\frac{P_k^2}{2m} + \frac{1}{2} m\omega_k^2 Q_k^2 \right) + V'(k)Q_k \right], \qquad (9.3)$$

where

$$V'(k) = \left[\frac{\partial V(q,Q_k)}{\partial Q_k} \right]_{Q_k=0}.$$

We shall be interested in the matrix elements of (9.3) in the basis set of the irreducible representations T_{2g}:

$$\mathcal{H}_{ij} = E_0 \delta_{ij} + \sum_k \left(\frac{P_k^2}{2m} + \frac{1}{2} m\omega_k^2 Q_k^2 \right) \delta_{ij} + \sum_k \langle i | V'(k) | j \rangle Q_k, \qquad (9.4)$$

in which i,j stand for any of the three functions ξ, η, ζ belonging to T_{2g}, and E_0 is the 3-fold degenerate eigenvalue of $\mathcal{H}_0(q,p)$.

Since the electronic eigenfunctions belong to the irreducible representation T_{2g}, the matrix element $\langle i | V'(k) | j \rangle$ will vanish unless $V'(k)$ transforms according to an irreducible representation contained in the symmetrized direct product $T_{2g} \times T_{2g}$; these are A_{1g}, E_g and T_{2g}. Moreover since $\mathcal{H}$ is an invariant under the operations of the symmetry group, $V'(k)$ and Q_k must transform according to the same irreducible representation. This leads to the conclusion that the normal modes of the nuclei which couple with the electronic state T_{2g}, belong to the irreducible representations α_{1g}, ε_g, τ_{2g} (we use Greek letters for nuclear modes). Of these, α_{1g} is the breathing mode and is of no significance since it can only shift the energy of an electronic state.

We now consider in further detail the coupling of an ε_g-nuclear mode with a T_{2g}-electronic state. According to the Wigner-Eckart theorem

$$\langle i | V'(k) | j \rangle = V \begin{pmatrix} T_{2g} & T_{2g} & \varepsilon_g \\ i & j & k \end{pmatrix} \langle T_{2g} \| V' \| T_{2g} \rangle, \qquad (9.5)$$

in which $\langle T_{2g} \| V' \| T_{2g} \rangle$ is a reduced matrix element. When the V coefficients (GRIFFITH, 1962) are inserted and the two members of ε_g are labeled by Q_u and Q_v, the Hamiltonian becomes

$$\mathcal{H} = A \begin{pmatrix} \frac{1}{2}Q_u - \frac{1}{2}\sqrt{3}Q_v & 0 & 0 \\ 0 & \frac{1}{2}Q_u + \frac{1}{2}\sqrt{3}Q_v & 0 \\ 0 & 0 & -Q_u \end{pmatrix} + [T + \frac{1}{2}m\omega^2(Q_u^2 + Q_v^2)]I, \qquad (9.6)$$

where we have set $E_0=0$, $T=(P_u^2+P_v^2)/2m$ and $\omega=\omega_u=\omega_v$; A is proportional to the reduced matrix and I is the unit matrix.

It is seen that in the basis set ξ, η, ζ, the Hamiltonian of the system is diagonal. If we put $\mathcal{H} = T + V$, then the three eigenvalues of V are

$$V_\xi = A\left(\frac{1}{2}Q_u - \frac{\sqrt{3}}{2}Q_v\right) + \frac{1}{2}m\omega^2(Q_u^2 + Q_v^2),$$

$$V_\eta = A\left(\frac{1}{2}Q_u + \frac{\sqrt{3}}{2}Q_v\right) + \frac{1}{2}m\omega^2(Q_u^2 + Q_v^2), \tag{9.7}$$

$$V_\zeta = -AQ_u \qquad\qquad + \frac{1}{2}m\omega^2(Q_u^2 + Q_v^2).$$

These are three parabaloids which differ from one another by a rotation of $2\pi/3$. The three minima are located at the same depth; thus V_ζ has a minimum at

$$Q_u^\zeta = \frac{A}{m\omega^2}, \qquad Q_v^\zeta = 0, \tag{9.8}$$

and at the minimum

$$V_\zeta^m = -\frac{A^2}{2m\omega^2} = E_{JT}(\varepsilon_g). \tag{9.9}$$

Reference to Fig. 9.1 shows that this represents the case in which the system is unstable against a tetragonal distortion in the z direction; in the same fashion V_ξ and V_η correspond to tetragonal distortions along x and y respectively.

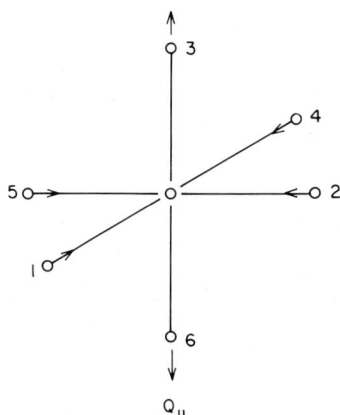

Fig. 9.1. The mode Q_u described by

$$Q_u = \frac{1}{\sqrt{12}}[2z_3 - 2z_6 - x_1 + x_4 - y_2 + y_5]$$

with respect to a right-handed coordinate system constructed at the equilibrium position of each ligand

We may summarize this discussion by saying that the Jahn-Teller effect associated with the coupling of an ε_g-vibrational mode to a T_{2g}-electronic state can produce a tetragonal distortion which lowers the symmetry of the configuration from O_h to D_{4h} and reduces the energy of the system by $A^2/2m\omega^2$. The original 3-fold degenerate electronic wavefunctions ξ, η, ζ are replaced by 3-fold degenerate vibronic wavefunctions which have the form of simple Born-Oppenheimer products.

The analysis of the $T_{2g} - \tau_{2g}$ coupling proceeds in an analogous fashion and leads to a trigonal distortion (D_{3d}); the presence of both couplings results in a competition between the two deformation modes. For a T_{2g} term in d^6 (ENGLEMAN, 1972)

$$\frac{E_{JT}(\varepsilon_g)}{E_{JT}(\tau_{2g})} = \frac{9}{4} \frac{\omega^2(\tau_{2g})}{\omega^2(\varepsilon_g)} \left[\left(1 - \frac{25}{27}\eta\right)\bigg/\left(1 - \frac{5}{9}\eta\right)\right] \tag{9.10}$$

with $\eta = 0.2 - 0.4$. For a highly covalent complex $E_{JT}(\varepsilon)/E_{JT}(\tau)$ can exceed unity.

It is now possible to state the Jahn-Teller hypothesis concerning hemoglobin (WEISSBLUTH, 1972): Oxyhemoglobin is in the low-spin state $t_{2g}^6\,{}^1A_{1g}$ with the Fe^{2+} ion in the plane of the heme. However, because of the delicate balance between Coulomb energy and cubic splitting, the high-spin $t_{2g}^4 e_g^2\,{}^5T_{2g}$) form is energetically close to the low-spin form. It is therefore postulated that there is a nonvanishing probability for thermal excitations from ${}^1A_{1g}$ to ${}^5T_{2g}$. The latter, on account of its degeneracy, is subject to a Jahn-Teller effect through inter-action with ε_g- and τ_{2g}-nuclear modes. It is assumed that because of the high covalency of oxyhemoglobin, the dominant coupling is $T_{2g} - \varepsilon_g$ which results in a tetragonal (D_{4h}) deformation mode along the x, y or z directions. Since the heme is a planar structure and sits in a pocket formed by the protein, it is ex-pected that the most likely deformation is in the z direction (perpendicular to the heme plane), as shown in Fig. 9.1. This deformation acting in conjunction with the constraints imposed by the protein is then assumed to lead to the displacement of Fe^{2+} from the heme plane and the simultaneous removal of the oxygen molecule. According to this view, then, it is energetically more favorable—by an amount $E_{JT}(\varepsilon_g)$—for an Fe^{2+} ion to be displaced from the heme plane once it gets into a high-spin state.

PERUTZ (1970) has discussed the stereochemical basis for the cooperative effects in the oxygenation of hemoglobin. Of central importance is the position of the Fe^{2+} ion relative to the heme plane. It is the change in the position of Fe^{2+} and the heme-linked histidine attached to it which initiates the complex series of conformational changes essential for cooperative behavior. More recently PERUTZ and TEN EYCK (1971) have reviewed the evidence leading to the viewpoint that in the deoxy form of hemoglobin the subunit contacts are stressed and that the salt bridges (Section 2.5) are necessary to maintain the deoxy quaternary conformation. The binding of oxygen is accompanied by rupture of the salt bridges, which allows the molecule to adopt a relaxed quaternary conformation. The question then arises as to the mechanism that "causes the quaternary struc-ture to switch from the oxy to the deoxy form once the constraints have been removed" (PERUTZ and TEN EYCK, 1971). The Jahn-Teller effect provides a possible mechanism, though it must be said that the evidence in support of such a hypothesis is not conclusive and for the time being at least, it must remain in the category of an interesting conjecture.

References

ABRAGAM, A., BLEANEY, R.: Electron Paramagnetic Resonance of Transition Ions. Oxford: Clarendon Press 1970.

ANTONINI, E., BRUNORI, M.: Hemoglobin. Ann. Rev. Biochem. **39**, 977—1042 (1970).

ANTONINI, E., BRUNORI, M.: Hemoglobin and Myoglobin in Their Reactions with Ligands. New York: American Elsevier 1971.

BALLHAUSEN, C. J.: Ligand Field Theory. New York: McGraw-Hill 1962.

BALLHAUSEN, C. J., GRAY, H. B.: Molecular Orbital Theory. New York: W. A. Benjamin 1965.

BEARDEN, A. J., DUNHAM, W. R.: Iron Electronic Configurations in Proteins: Studies by Mossbauer Spectroscopy. In: Structure and Bonding, Vol. 8, pp. 1—52. Berlin-Heidelberg-New York: Springer 1970.

BLUMBERG, W. E., PEISACH, J.: The Ligands of Low-Spin Ferric Compounds of Hemoglobin A. In: Genetical, Functional, and Physical Studies of Hemoglobins, T. Arends, B. Bemski and R. L. Nagel, Eds. Basel: S. Karger 1971.

BOLTON, W., PERUTZ, M. F.: Three Dimensional Fourier Synthesis of Horse Deoxyhaemoglobin at 2.8 Å Resolution. Nature **228**, 551—552 (1970).

BRACKETT, G. C., RICHARDS, P. L., CAUGHEY, W. S., WICKMAN, H. H.: Far-Infrared Magnetic Resonance in Fe(III) and Mn(III) Porphyrins, Myoglobin, Hemoglobin, Ferrichrome A and Fe(III) Dithiocarbamates. J. Chem. Phys. **54**, 4383—4401 (1971).

BRADFORD, E., MARSHALL, W.: Mossbauer Absorption in the Presence of Electron Spin Relaxation. Proc. Phys. Soc. **87**, 731—747 (1966).

DALZIEL, K., O'BRIEN, J. R. P.: The Kinetics of Deoxygenation of Human Hemoglobin. Biochem. J. **78**, 236—245 (1961).

DEBRUNNER, P. G.: Mossbauer Spectroscopy of Biomolecules. In: Spectroscopic Approaches to Biomolecular Conformation, D. W. Urry, Ed. Am. Med. Assoc. Press 1970.

DICKERSON, R. E., GEIS, I.: The Structure and Action of Proteins. New York: Harper and Row 1969.

DYSON, F. J.: The Future of Physics. Physics Today **23**, 23—28 (1970).

EDSALL, J. T., FLORY, P. F., KENDREW, J. C., LIQUORI, A. M., NEMETHY, G., RAMACHANDRAN, G. N., SCHERAGA, H. A.: A Proposal of Standard Conventions and Nomenclature for the Description of Polypeptide Conformations. J. molec. Biol. **15**, 399—407 (1966).

EDSALL, J. T., WYMAN, J.: Biophysical Chemistry. New York: Academic Press 1958.

EICHER, H., TRAUTWEIN, A.: Electronic Structure of Ferrous Iron in Hemoglobin Inferred from Mossbauer Measurements. J. Chem. Phys. **52**, 932—934 (1970).

ENGLMAN, R.: The Jahn-Teller Effect in Molecules and Crystals. New York: Wiley-Interscience 1972.

FLETCHER, J. E., SPECTOR, A. A., ASHBROOK, J. D.: Analysis of Macromolecule-Ligand Binding by Determination of Stepwise Equilibrium Constants. Biochemistry **9**, 4580—4587 (1970).

FRAUENFELDER, H.: The Mossbauer Effect. New York: W. A. Benjamin 1962.

FRUTON, J. S., SIMMONDS, S.: General Biochemistry. New York: John Wiley 1958.

GEORGE, P., BEETLESTONE, J., GRIFFITH, J. S.: Ferrihemoprotein Hydroxides: A Correlation Between Magnetic and Spectroscopic Properties. Rev. mod. Phys. **36**, 441—458 (1964).

GIBSON, Q. H.: The Reaction of Oxygen with Hemoglobin and the Kinetic Basis of the Effect of Salt on Binding of Oxygen. J. Biol. Chem. **245**, 3285—3288 (1970).

GIBSON, Q. H.: The Contribution of the α and β Chains to the Kinetics of Oxygen Binding to and Dissociation from Hemoglobin. Proc. Nat. Acad. Sci. (Wash.) **70**, 1—4 (1973).

GIBSON, J. F., INGRAM, D. J. E.: Electron Resonance Studies of Hemoglobin Azide and Hydroxide Derivatives. Nature **180**, 29—30 (1957).

GIBSON, J. F., INGRAM, D. J. E., SCHONLAND, D.: Magnetic Resonance of Different Ferric Complexes. Disc. Farad. Soc. **26**, 72—80 (1958).

GREENWOOD, N. N., GIBB, T. C.: Mossbauer Spectroscopy. London: Chapman and Hall 1971.

GRIFFITH, J. S.: On the Magnetic Properties of Some Haemoglobin Complexes. Proc. Roy. Soc. (London) **235A**, 23—36 (1956).

GRIFFITH, J. S.: On the Stabilities of Transition Metal Complexes—I. Theory of the Energies. J. Inorg. Chem. **2**, 1—10 (1956a).

GRIFFITH, J. S.: Theory of Electron Resonance in Ferrihaemoglobin Azide. Nature **180**, 30—31 (1957).

GRIFFITH, J. S.: The Theory of Transition Metal Ions. Cambridge University Press 1961.

GRIFFITH, J. S.: The Irreducible Tensor Method for Molecular Symmetry Groups. Englewood Cliffs, N.J.: Prentice-Hall 1962.

GRIFFITH, J. S.: Theory of EPR in Low-Spin Ferric Haemoproteins. Molec. Phys. **21**, 135—139 (1971).

GUIDOTTI, G.: The Functional Properties of the Subunits of Hemoglobin. In: Genetical, Functional, and Physical Studies of Hemoglobin, T. Arends, G. Bemski and R. L. Nagel, Eds. pp. 113—122. Basel: S. Karger 1971.

HAM, F. S.: Jahn-Teller Effects in Electron Paramagnetic Resonance. In: Electron Paramagnetic Resonance, S. Geschwind, Ed. New York: Plenum Press 1972.

HARRIS-LOEW, G. M.: An Analysis of the Electron Spin Resonance of Low Spin Ferric Heme Compounds. Biophys. J. **10**, 196—212 (1970).

HELCKE, G. A., INGRAM, D. J. E., SLADE, E. F.: Electron Resonance Studies of Haemoglobin Derivatives IV. Line-Width and g-value Measurements of Acid-Met Myoglobin and of Met Myoglobin Azide Derivatives. Proc. Roy. Soc. **B169**, 275—288 (1968).

HEWITT, J. A., KILMARTIN, J. V., TEN EYCK, L. F., PERUTZ, M. F.: Noncooperativity of the $\alpha\beta$ Dimer in the Reaction of Hemoglobin with Oxygen. Proc. Nat. Acad. Sci. (Wash.) **69**, 203—207 (1972).

HOARD, J. L.: Some Aspects of Heme Stereochemistry. In: Structural Chemistry and Molecular Biology, A. Rich and N. Davidson, Eds. San Francisco: W. H. Freeman 1968.

HOARD, J. L.: Stereochemistry of Hemes and Other Metalloporphyrins. Science **174**, 1295—1302 (1971).

HOPFIELD, J. J.: The Relation Between Structure, Cooperativity, and Spectra in a Model of Hemoglobin Action (in press, 1973).

HOPFIELD, J. J., SHULMAN, R. G., OGAWA, S.: An Allosteric Model of Hemoglobin: I. Kinetics. J. molec. Biol. **61**, 425—443 (1971).

IIZUKA, T., KOTANI, M.: Analysis of a Thermal Equilibrium Phenomenon Between High-Spin and Low-Spin States of Ferrimyoglobin Azide. Biochim. Biophys. Acta **154**, 417—419 (1968).

IIZUKA, T., YONETANI, T.: Spin Changes in Hemoproteins. Advanc. Biophys. **1**, 157—182 (1970).

INGALLS, R.: Electric-Field Gradient Tensor in Ferrous Compounds. Phys. Rev. **133**, A 787—795 (1964).

JUDD, B. R.: Operator Techniques in Atomic Spectroscopy. New York: McGraw-Hill 1963.

KAMIMURA, H., MIZUHASHI, S.: Magnetic Anisotropy due to Dynamical Jahn-Teller Effect in $d\varepsilon^1$ and $d\varepsilon^5$ Ions. J. appl. Phys. **39**, 684—686 (1968).

KELLETT, G. L., GUTFREUND, H.: Reactions of Haemoglobin Dimers After Ligand Dissociation. Nature **227**, 921—926 (1970).

KONIG, E., KREMER, S.: Temperature Dependence of the $^5T_2 - {}^1A_1$ Energy Separation at the Ground-State Crossover in $[Fe^{II} - N_6]$ Complexes. Chem. Phys. Let. **8**, 812—313 (1971).

KOSHLAND, D. E. Jr., NEMETHY, G., FILMER, D.: Comparison of Experimental Binding Data and Theoretical Models in Proteins Containing Subunits. Biochemistry **5**, 365—385 (1966).

KOSTER, A. S.: Electronic State of Iron in Hemoglobin, Myoglobin, and Derivatives, as Inferred from X-Ray Fluorescence Spectra. J. Chem. Phys. **56**, 3161—3164 (1972).

KOSTER, G. F., DIMMOCK, J. O., WHEELER, R. G., STATZ, H.: Properties of the Thirty-Two Point Groups. Cambridge: MIT Press 1963.

KOTANI, M.: Theoretical Study on the Effective Magnetic Moments of Some Hemoproteins. Progr. Theoret. Phys. (Kyoto) Suppl. **17**, 4—13 (1961).

KOTANI, M.: Electronic Structure and Magnetic Properties of Hemoproteins, Particularly of Hemoglobins. Advanc. Chem. Phys. **7**, 159—181 (1964a).

KOTANI, M.: Note on the Electronic Interaction Between Imidazole and Iron in Heme. Biopolym. Symp. **1**, 67—73 (1964b).

KOTANI, M.: Paramagnetic Properties and Electronic Structure of Iron in Heme Proteins. Advanc. Quant. Chem. **4**, 227—266 (1968).

KOTANI, M., MORIMOTO, H.: EPR Studies on Single Crystals of Myoglobin and Myoglobin Fluoride. In: Magnetic Resonance in Biological Systems, A. Ehrenberg, B. G. Malmstrom and T. Vanngard, Eds. New York: Pergamon 1967.

LANG, G.: Biological Applications of Magnetism. J. appl. Phys. **38**, 915—922 (1967).

LANG, G.: Mossbauer Spectroscopy of Haem Proteins. Quart. Rev. Biophys. **3**, 1—60 (1970).

LANG, G., MARSHALL, W.: Mossbauer Effect in Some Hemoglobin Compounds. Proc. Phys. Soc. **87**, 3—34 (1966).

LEHNINGER, A. L.: Biochemistry. New York: Worth Publishers 1970.

LINDSTROM, T. R., HO, C.: Functional Nonequivalence of α and β Hemes in Human Adult Hemoglobin. Proc. Nat. Acad. Sci. (Wash.) **69**, 1707—1710 (1972).

LOW, W.: Paramagnetic Resonance in Solids. New York: Academic Press 1960.

MAHLER, H. R., CORDES, E. H.: Biological Chemistry. New York: Harper and Row 1967.

MALING, J. E., WEISSBLUTH, M.: The Application of Mossbauer Spectroscopy to the Study of Iron in Heme Protein. In: Solid-State Biophysics, S. J. Wyard, Ed. New York: McGraw-Hill 1969.

McCONNELL, H. M.: Spin-Label Studies of Cooperative Oxygen Binding to Hemoglobin. Ann. Rev. Biochem. **40**, 227—236 (1971).

McCONNELL H. M., McFARLAND, B. G.: Physics and Chemistry of Spin Labels. Quart. Rev. Biophys. **3**, 91—136 (1970).

MIZUHASHI, S.: Anisotropy of g-Values in Low-Spin Ferrihaemoglobin Azide. J. Phys. Soc. Japan **26**, 468—492 (1969).

MONOD, J., WYMAN, J., CHANGEUX, J.-P.: On the Nature of Allosteric Transitions: A Plausible Model. J. molec. Biol. **12**, 88—118 (1965).

MORIMOTO, H., KOTANI, M.: Fluorine Superhyperfine Structure in EPR Spectra of the Single Crystal of the Myoglobin Fluoride. Biochim. Biophys. Acta **126**, 176—178 (1966).

MORIMOTO, H., LEHMANN, H., PERUTZ, M. F.: Molecular Pathology of Human Haemoglobin: Stereochemical Interpretation of Abnormal Oxygen Affinities. Nature **232**, 408—413 (1971).

MUIRHEAD, H., COX, J. M., MAZZARELLA, L., PERUTZ, M. F.: Structure and Function of Hemoglobin III. A Three-Dimensional Fourier Synthesis of Human Deoxyhemoglobin at 5.5 Å Resolution. J. molec. Biol. **28**, 117—156 (1967).

MUIRHEAD, H., GREER, J.: Three-dimensional Fourier Synthesis of Human Deoxyhaemoglobin at 3.5 Å Resolution. Nature **228**, 516—519 (1970).

OGATA, R. T., McCONNELL, H. M.: The Binding of Spin-Labeled Triphosphate to Hemoglobin. Cold Spr. Harb. Symp. Quant. Biol. **36**, 325—335 (1971).

OGATA, R. T., McCONNELL, H. M.: Mechanism of Cooperative Oxygen Binding in Hemoglobin. Proc. Nat. Acad. Sci. (Wash.) **69**, 335—339 (1972).

OGAWA, S., SHULMAN, R. G., YAMANE, T.: High Resolution Nuclear Magnetic Resonance Spectra of Hemoglobin I. The Cyanide Complexes of α and β Chains. J. molec. Biol. **70** 291—300 (1972).

OGAWA, S., SHULMAN, R. G., FUJIWARA, M., YAMANE, T.: High Resolution Nuclear Magnetic Resonance Spectra of Hemoglobin II. Ligated Tetramers. J. molec. Biol. **70**, 301—313 (1972a).

OGAWA, S., SHULMAN, R. G.: High Resolution Nuclear Magnetic Resonance Spectra of Hemoglobin III. The Half-Ligated State and Allosteric Interactions. J. molec. Biol. **70**, 315—336 (1972).

OHNO, K., TANABE, Y., SASAKI, F.: Simple Molecular Orbital Calculations on the Electronic Structure of Iron-Porphyrin Complexes. Theoret. Chim. Acta (Berl.) **1**, 378—392 (1963).

PAULING, L.: The Electronic Structure of Haemoglobin. London: Butterworths 1949.

PAULING, L.: Nature of the Iron-Oxygen Bond in Oxyhemoglobin. Nature **203**, 182—183 (1964).

PAULING, L., CORYELL, C. D.: The Magnetic Properties and Structure of Hemoglobin, Oxyhemoglobin and Carbonmonoxyhemoglobin. Proc. Nat. Acad. Sci. (Wash.) **22**, 210—216 (1936).

PAULING, L., COREY, R., BRANSON, H.: The Structure of Proteins: Two Hydrogen-Bonded Helical Configurations of the Polypeptide Chain. Proc. Nat. Acad. Sci. (Wash.) **37**, 205—211 (1951).

PEISACH, J., BLUMBERG, W. E.: The Specific Compounds Formed During the Reversible and Irreversible Denaturation of Hemoglobin and its Constituent Chains. In: Genetical, Functional and Physical Studies of Hemoglobin, T. Arends, G. Bemski and R. L. Nagel, Eds. Basel: S. Karger 1971.

PEISACH, A., BLUMBERG, W. E., WITTENBERG, B. A., WITTENBERG, J. G., KAMPA, L.: Hemoglobin A: An Electron Paramagnetic Resonance Study of the Effects of Interchain Contacts on the Heme

Symmetry of High-Spin and Low-Spin Derivatives of Ferric Alpha Chains. Proc. Nat. Acad. Sci. (Wash.) **63**, 934—939 (1969).

PEISACH, J., BLUMBERG, W. E., OGAWA, S., RACHMILEWITZ, E. A., OLTZIK, R.: The Effects of Protein Conformation on the Heme Symmetry in High-Spin Ferric Heme Proteins as Studied by Electron Paramagnetic Resonance. J. biol. Chem. **246**, 3342—3355 (1971).

PERUTZ, M. F.: The Hemoglobin Molecule. Scientific American **211**, 64—76 (1964).

PERUTZ, M. F.: The Haemoglobin Molecule. Proc. Roy. Soc. **B173**, 113—140 (1969a).

PERUTZ, M. F.: X-ray Analysis, Structure and Function of Enzymes. Europ. J. Biochem. **8**, 455—466 (1969b).

PERUTZ, M. F.: Stereochemistry of Cooperative Effects in Haemoglobin. Nature **228**, 726—739 (1970).

PERUTZ, M. F.: Nature of Haem-Haem Interaction. Nature **237**, 495—499 (1972).

PERUTZ, M. F., MUIRHEAD, H., COX, J. M., GOAMAN, L. C. G., MATHEWS, F. S., MCGANDY, E. L., WEBB, L. E.: Three-dimensional Fourier Synthesis of Horse Oxyhaemoglobin at 2.8 Å Resolution: (1) X-ray Analysis. Nature **219**, 29—32 (1968a).

PERUTZ, M. F., MUIRHEAD, H., COX, J. M. GOAMAN, L. C. G.: Three-dimensional Fourier Synthesis of Horse Oxyhaemoglobin at 2.8 Å Resolution: II The Atomic Model. Nature **219**, 131—139 (1968b).

PERUTZ, M. F., TEN EYCK, L. F.: Stereochemistry of Cooperative Effects in Hemoglobin. Cold. Spr. Harb. Symp. Quant. Biol. **36**, 295—310 (1971).

ROTENBERG, M., BIVINS, R., METROPOLIS, N., WOOTEN, J. K., Jr.: The 3-j and 6-j Symbols. Cambridge, Mass.: The Technology Press MIT 1959.

SAROFF, H. A., MINTON, A. P.: The Hill Plot and the Energy of Interaction in Hemoglobin. Science **175**, 1253—1255 (1972).

SCHELER, W., SCHOFFA, G., JUNG, F.: Lichtabsorption und Paramagnetische Suszeptibilität bei Derivaten des Pferde- und Chironomas-Methämoglobins sowie des Pferde-Metmyoglobins. Biochem. Z. **329**, 232—246 (1957).

SCHOFFA, G.: Magnetic Susceptibilities and the Chemical Bond in Hemoproteins. Advanc. Chem. Phys. **7**, 182—198 (1964).

SLATER, J. C.: Quantum Theory of Atomic Structure. New York: McGraw-Hill 1960.

SMITH, D. W., WILLIAMS, R. J. P.: The Spectra of Ferric Haems and Haemoproteins. In: Structure and Bonding, Vol. 7, pp. 1—45. Berlin-Heidelberg-New York: Springer 1970.

STRYER, L., KENDREW, J. C., WATSON, H. C.: The Mode of Attachment of the Azide Ion to Sperm Whale Metmyoglobin. J. molec. Biol. **8**, 96—104 (1964).

STURGE, M. D.: The Jahn-Teller Effect in Solids. Solid State Physics **20**, 91—211 (1967).

SZABO, A., KARPLUS, M.: A Mathematical Model for Structure-Function Relations in Hemoglobin. J. molec. Biol. **72**, 163—197 (1972).

TANABE, Y., SUGANO, S.: On the Absorption Spectra of Complex Ions II. J. Phys. Soc. Japan **9**, 766—779 (1954).

TASAKI, A., OTSUKA, J., KOTANI, M.: Magnetic Susceptibility Measurements on Hemoproteins Down to 4.2° K. Biochim. Biophys. Acta **140**, 284—290 (1967).

THOMPSON, C. J.: Models for Hemoglobin and Allosteric Enzymes. Biopolym. **6**, 1101—1118 (1968).

TRAUTWEIN, A., EICHER, H., MEYER, A., ALFSEN, A., WAKS, M., ROSA, J., BEAUZARD, Y.: Modification of the Electronic Structure of Ferrous Iron in Hemoglobin by Ligandation and by Alterations of the Protein Structure Inferred from Mossbauer Experiments. J. chem. Phys. **53**, 963—967 (1970).

WATANABE, H.: Operator Methods in Ligand Field Theory. Englewood Cliffs: Prentice Hall 1966.

WEISS, J. J.: Nature of the Iron-Oxygen Bond in Oxyhemoglobin. Nature **202**, 83—84 (1964).

WEISSBLUTH, M.: The Physics of Hemoglobin. In: Structure and Bonding, Vol. 2, pp. 1—125. Berlin-Heidelberg-New York: Springer 1967.

WEISSBLUTH, M.: Relaxation Effects in the Mossbauer Spectra of Hemoglobin. In: Genetical, Functional and Physical Studies of Hemoglobin, T. Arends, G. Bemski, and R. L. Nagel, Eds. Basel: S. Karger 1971.

WEISSBLUTH, M.: The Jahn-Teller Effect in Hemoglobin. J. theoret. Biol. **35**, 597—600 (1972).

WEISSBLUTH, M., MALING, J.: Interpretation of Quadrupole Splittings and Isomer Shifts in Hemoglobin. J. chem. Phys. **47**, 4166—4172 (1967).

WERTHEIM, G. K.: Mossbauer Effect: Principles and Applications. New York: Academic Press 1964.

WINTER, M. R. C., JOHNSON, C. E., LANG, G., WILLIAMS, R. J. P.: Mossbauer Spectroscopy of Haemoglobin Derivatives. Biochim. Biophys. Acta **263**, 515—534 (1972).

WITTENBERG, J. B., WITTENBERG, B. A., PEISACH, J., BLUMBERG, W. E.: On the State of the Iron and the Nature of the Ligand in Oxyhemoglobin. Proc. Nat. Acad. Sci. (Wash.) **67**, 1846—1853 (1970).

WÜTHRICH, K.: Structural Studies of Hemes and Hemoproteins by Nuclear Magnetic Resonance Spectroscopy. In: Structure and Bonding, Vol. 8, pp. 53—121. Berlin-Heidelberg-New York: Springer 1970.

WYMAN, J., Jr.: Linked Functions and Reciprocal Effects in Hemoglobin: A Second Look. Advanc. Protein Chem. **19**, 223—286 (1964).

WYMAN, J., Jr.: Allosteric Linkage. J. Am. chem. Soc. **89**, 2202—2218 (1967).

WYMAN, J., Jr.: Regulation in Macromolecules as Illustrated by Haemoglobin. Quart. Rev. Biophys. **1**, 35—80 (1968).

ZERNER, M., GOUTERMAN, M., KOBAYASHI, H.: Porphyrins VIII. Extended Hückel Calculations on Iron Complexes. Theoret. Chim. Acta (Berl.) **6**, 363—400 (1966).

ZIMAN, J. M.: Principles of the Theory of Solids. Cambridge University Press 1965.

Subject Index

Molecular Biology, Biochemistry and Biophysics